Spirit Centered Wholeness

Beyond the Psychology of Self

Spirit Centered Wholeness

Beyond the Psychology of Self

edited by

H. Newton Malony, Michele Papen-Daniels
& Howard Clinebell

Studies in the Psychology of Religion
Volume 2

The Edwin Mellen Press
Lewiston/Queenston

Library of Congress Cataloging-in-Publication Data

Malony, H. Newton
Spirit-centered wholeness beyond the psychology of self.

(Studies in the psychology of religion ; v. 2)
Bibliography : p.
Includes index.
1. Spirituality. 2. Psychology, Religious.
I. Title. II. Series.
BL624.M32 1988 291.2'2 87-25028
ISBN 0-88946-246-1

This is volume 2 in the continuing series
Studies in the Psychology of Religion
Volume 2 ISBN 0-88946-246-1
SPR Series ISBN 0-88946-247-X

For information contact:

The Edwin Mellen Press
P.O.Box 450
Lewiston, New York
USA 14092

The Edwin Mellen Press
P.O. Box 67
Queenston, Ontario
CANADA L0S 1L0

Printed in the United States of America

Contributors

Moreen Kamiki Cutter Bratt is Instructor in Art History, the University of La Verne, La Verne, California.

Howard Cinebell is Professor of Pastoral Counseling at the School of Theology, Claremont, California. He is the director of the Institute for Religion and Wholeness.

John B. Cobb, Jr. is Professor of Theology and director of the Institute for Process Studies at the School of Theology, Claremont, California.

Nelson E. Haggerson, is Professor of Education, Arizona State University, Tempe, Arizona.

Catherine Keller is Assistant Professor of Religion at Xavier University, Cincinnati, Ohio.

H. Newton Malony is Professor and Director of Programs in the Integration of Psychology and Theology, The Graduate School of Psychology, Fuller Theological Seminary, Pasadena, California.

Donald E. Miller is Professor in the School of Religion, the University of Southern California, Los Angeles, California.

David S. Pacini is Associate Professor of Historical Theology, Candler School of Theology, Emory University, Atlanta, Georgia.

Michele Papen-Daniels is Assistant Professor, California State University, Bakersfield, California.

John E. Roberts is a psychotherapist in private practice, Santa Monica, California.

Orlo Strunk is Professor Emeritus of Pastoral Counseling (Retired), the School of Theology, Boston University, Boston, Massachusetts.

TABLE OF CONTENTS

Foreword

The theologian Paul Tillich reportedly said that everyone was "centered in self." Such a statement poses both the possibility and the problem of such a volume as this.

The theme of this volume is spirit-, not self-, centered wholeness. Is it possible that in understanding the kind of wholeness which is centered in "spirit" we will discover the "self"? This is the possibility that we hope will prove true because we are convinced that the spirit is at the core of selfhood. In tripartite language, we are convinced that the self is composed of body, mind, AND spirit. Of course, this assertion is not new with us. We are indebted to the heritage of the ages. Our debt is to Plato, to Isaiah, to the Buddha, to St. Paul, to philosophers such as Kant and to theologians such as Berkouwer. Tillich is not a lonely voice crying in the wilderness, nor are we.

The statement that humans are "spiritual beings" is heard from many voices today apart from those in religious circles. These voices range from the transpersonal psychologists to the physicists. Of course, there are those empiricists who still continue the age-old expedition of seeking to find the biological location of spirit. When they do not find it, they say that spirit does not exist. They are impatient with the rest of us who say that not only does spirit exist but that it is the very essence of what being human means. We feel the location of spirit is far less important than its function and its dynamic power. We know no better solution to this issue than that given by Descartes who simply said that spirit IS and that it operates by laws that cannot be reduced to matter.

SPIRIT-centered wholeness, then, is the bold topic around which these essays are addressed. Each of them explores the conviction that spirit is the central fact of human existence and that the explication of the meaning of that conviction is of extreme importance to human wholeness and well-being. To be centered in self means to be centered in spirit. To ignore this truth or to live apart from it is to exist at a less than fully human level. The possibility that these ideas will enliven and enlighten your understanding of this central fact is the hope of this volume.

There is no escaping the fact that each of us views the world through our own eyes. We have no choice. Perhaps that is what Tillich meant by his comment that humans are centered in self. Without question, this is what Einstein implied in his theory of relativity. The world centers around us; our perceptions, our judgments, our fears, our hopes.

We said that Tillich's comment about everyone being "centered in self" but not necessarily being "self-centered" poses a problem alongside the real possibility that such a volume as this will stimulate understanding and inspire fulfilled living. The greatest temptation of life is that of narcissism and pride that blocks wholeness. To become self-centered is to become prideful and closed to freeing insight from life, God, others, and the divine Spirit. A discussion on spirit-centered wholeness runs the danger of seeming to encourage selfishness and elitism.

Scholarship often breeds pride in its own achievements and disdain for the "unenlightened." Sometimes this leads to an unwillingness to learn from the wisdom of those outside the academy. Our understanding is that spirit-centeredness is at its heart self-transcending. This is precisely the orientation that moves one away from self-absorption and narcissism.

Nevertheless, there is a temptation to become prideful about becoming more whole by becoming more spirit-centered, as if spirit-centeredness was like body building or scholastic achievement. The elitism of sanctified persons is well-known. William James wrote about the dangers of too much saintliness. He was not the first, nor the last, to note this problem. Reading these essays as if they were "how to" instructions on "getting it all-together with the spirit" is, we recognize, a potential problem with volumes such as this.

Our intent, however, is to avoid self-centeredness. Our hope would be to by-pass that problem in favor of the possibility that we may, in truth, contribute to a deeper awareness of what spirit-centered living can mean to others as well as ourselves.

Whereas one's body and one's mind are one's own, spirit seems to refer to something bigger than oneself. Jung's "collective unconscious" referred to a depth in the self that was larger than personal experience. Immanuel Kant contended that the conscience or the sense of moral obligation was each person's connection with the will of God. St. Paul put it well when he wrote, "God's Spirit joins himself to our spirit to declare that we are God's children" (Romans 8:16, TEV).

Some readers will be disappointed with the "headiness" of these essays. They are not meant for bedtime reading, as one would read a novel. They are intended to stimulate reflection, introspective dialogue and further exploration.

They are among those papers which were originally presented as the first theory-building conference of the Institute for Religion and Wholeness, an interdisciplinary group of seekers sponsored by the School of Theology at Claremont, California. We have chosen these essays from among the 19 that were delivered there as representative of the creative thinking that was done at this conference in the spring of 1983.

Other readers will be dismayed by the heterogeneity of the ideas. It is possible to miss the unifying motif that runs through them all. Each of these scholars wrote on the meaning of spirit-centered wholeness. Their ideas, however, reflect the varied disciplines from which they came and/or the concerns which were important to them at that time. We suggest that such variety makes for the richness of insights around a complex, many-faceted theme.

Understanding what it means to be "spirit-centered" and "whole" is a relatively unexplored territory. Certainly many more voices than these need to be heard before these crucial concepts will be fully understood. We trust that there will be many readers who will find these essays stimulating and provocative in part BECAUSE of their diversity rather than in spite of it. We hope there will be something inviting here for every serious student of wholeness of spirit.

These essays follow a model in their organization. It is presented in the first essay by Howard Clinebell. His flower model, with spiritual wholeness at the core and the other five dimensions as the petals, is the organizing idea around which the other essays are presented. Clinebell suggests that a living, growing "flower" is an appropriate paradigm around which to think about spiritual wholeness because of its natural development and its stages of becoming. Spiritual wholeness is not a given or a stated goal. It is a journey and a process. It grows. It develops. These essays suggest some ways to enable this growth in ourselves and others.

The beauty of spirit-centered wholeness, however, is dependent on the balanced development of each of its petals. Here is where the several dimensions of wholeness come in, according to Clinebell. He mentions these dimensions: the environmental, the relational, the institutional, the psychological, the physical and the spiritual. All of these play a part in making the blossom radiant, balanced, and beautiful. The integrating center of the flower is termed "spiritual wholeness." But there can be no spiritual wholeness without the spirit permeating the physical, psychological, institutional, relational and environmental dimensions of life.

Two essays are included under the environmental dimension of spiritual wholeness. David Pacini's essay on "Religion and wholeness in the shadow of modernity" takes the reader on a philosophical and historical trek back through the last several hundred years of western history and grounds one in a depth understanding of how one can speak of spiritual wholeness in the modern world. It is an awesome and somewhat fearsome journey. His essay is followed by Catherine Keller's analysis of contemporary culture in light of the relationships between the sexes and the importance of the feminine perspective on wholeness. Her essay is entitled "Wholeness and all the king's men."

The relational dimension includes two essays, also. Newton Malony's essay on "Whole holiness: holy wholeness" deals with the issue of ethics and wholeness. His contention is that there is no wholeness apart from a concern for others. Moreen Kamiki Cutter Bratt, an art-historian, discusses the ancient Minoan culture whose artifacts reflect an androgynous way of life in which individuality and potentiality were affirmed. Her essay is entitled "Dancing with Notitia; the spirit-centered female core of knowledge."

The psychological dimension includes two essays on individual experience and personal development. John Roberts discusses the essential ingredients of Vedic philosophy as they relate to this view of what it means to be fully human. His article is entitled "Wholeness: the perspectives of Indian idealism." Orlo Strunk, writing from within the Christian tradition, presents a model for inner growth that is grounded in meditation and contemplation in an essay entitled "Solitude, silence and personhood."

Donald Miller, a sociologist of religion, writes about the importance of institutions and community in his article "Religious community and human wholeness." His essay reflects the institutional dimension. He presents a positive, yet reflective understanding of the importance of social structures in cultivating or diminishing wholeness. The other institutional essay is entitled "Spirit-centered wholeness in education." Herein, Haggerson discusses the issue of a curriculum based on the viewpoint that human nature is essentially transcendent. He emphasizes the value of experience over information.

Finally, theologian John Cobb concludes the volume with a crucial essay on "Wholeness centered in spirit." He emphasizes the ideal toward which both spirit and wholeness pull human beings. He notes that while, on the one hand, spirit-centered wholeness is considered as an achievement toward which persons should aspire, on the other hand, it is a gift that results from trust in a transcendent power which cannot be controlled or manipulated.

The reader will quickly note that we have not included a section on the "physical" dimension. This is not because we did not consider the bodily dimensions of spirit-centered wholeness important. We felt, however, that of all the dimensions that were considered, the physical had been most discussed in recent times. The intentional omission of an essay on the physical serves to highlight the other less well considered aspects.

Is such a volume as this necessary or valuable? We think it is. There is no question but that we in the Institute of Religion and Wholeness have depended on ideas such as these to stimulate, guide, and nurture our work. We think the insights presented here are valuable even though they are, by no means, exhaustive or complete. We hope that they will be valued as stimuli for personal explorations and that readers will seek to go beyond them. We offer them to others in this spirit. Our trust is that there will be many more possibilities than problems in the reading of this volume.

H. Newton Malony
Michele Papen-Daniels
Howard Clinebell
Epiphany Season 1987

The Six Dimensions of Wholeness Centered in Spirit

Howard Clinebell

INTRODUCTION: This paper will present the conceptual model of Spirit-centered wholeness which I find most useful in the teaching and practice of pastoral counseling and psychotherapy. It will reflect on these themes:

- --The nature of six interdependent dimensions of human wholeness--physical, psychological, interpersonal, institutional, ecological and spirit--and how they interrelate.
- --The central, integrating dynamic of the spirit-dimension.
- --Some criteria for identifying wholeness-nurturing (vs wholeness-diminishing) beliefs and practices in the spiritual dimension.

Finally, I will illustrate my discussion with clinical observations derived from working with persons addicted to alcohol. Because I have discussed methods of facilitating spiritual wholeness at some length elsewhere, I will not deal with methodology issues here. (Clinebell, 1979, Chapters 3 & 4).

I. THE SIX DIMENSIONS OF WHOLENESS

(1) HEALING AND ENLIVENING OUR BODIES

The foundational dimension of wholeness is the wholeness of our physical organism. The degree of wholeness in this dimension, as in the other five, is on a continuum from debilitating pathology to high level wellness. Physical health or wholeness is more than the <u>absence</u> of diagnosable pathology. It is the <u>presence</u> of the positive wellness characterized by a vital, enlivened body. There are many degrees of wellness just as there are many degrees of sickness. As the body therapies and research on psychophysiological problems make clear, whatever diminishes physical wholeness tends to lessen mental and spiritual wholeness, and vice versa. But there are many striking exceptions to this general tendency--persons who are able to transcend physical illnesses and handicaps, to achieve high levels of mental and spiritual creativity. (The interrelationship between physical and spiritual wholeness obviously is very complex.)

A basic alienation that diminishes the wholeness of many people is an inner estrangement from their bodies. Alexander Lowen observes:

> Personality is much broader than consciousness . . . It is an expression of the total being: of its physical vitality, of its muscular coordination, of its inner harmony and outward grace. The magnetism of a personality is . . .the radiance of an alive body in which the mental and physical aspects reflect each other. (1968, p. 172)
>
> The ego depends for its sense of identity upon the perception of the body. If the body is charged and responsive . . .the ego image will be grounded in body image. (1967, pp. 37-38)

The foundational goals of wholeness-oriented counseling, psychotherapy, and medical practice must be the healing of disease, but all these disciplines should go beyond repair to help people maximize their level of positive wellness. This involves enabling persons to free their bodies from chronic self-stressing, constrictions of breathing and muscular tensions so that the whole organism can experience increased vitality.

By concentrating almost exclusively on healing psyches, traditional psychotherapies have joined with dualistic theologies in helping to maintain the inner split between our minds and spirits, on the one hand, and our bodies, on the other. Wholeness-oriented therapies seek to enable people to awaken their dulled senses, recover sensuous aliveness in their whole bodies, and thus regain some of the wonder, spontaneity and playfulness they have buried under lopsided rationality and overcontrol. When this happens, people often reclaim their "forsaken body with all the fervor of the lost child finding its loving mother" [or father] (Lowen, 1967, p. 231)

The relation of the enhancement of physical wholeness to increased spiritual wholeness often is crucial. Affirming our bodies' humanness may help to liberate our spiritual potentialities. We may move to what Sam Keen calls an "Incarnate existence" in which we experience the sacred <u>in</u> the so-called secular, and thereby gain a new respect not only for our bodies but for all living things. Enlivening religion, as Keen makes clear, must be danced and not just believed. (Keen, 1970, concluding essay).

(2) HEALING AND ENLIVENING OUR MINDS

The second dimension of wholeness is the wholeness of our minds. Increasingly wholeness in this crucial aspect of our humanity involves developing our many-faceted personality capacities including our intellectual resources. Here are some of the directions of growth toward greater psychic wholeness:

--Increasing awareness of one's total self, including the depths of one's psyche.

--growing awareness of and respect for reality.

--increasing self-identity, self-support and self-esteem.

--increasing intellectual competence, creativity, and playfulness.

--greater freshness of perception and richness of feelings (both joy and pain).

--a widening openness to newness.

--an increasing development of one's androgynous psychological resources.

--a growing enjoyment of living in one's present experience, enriched by one's past and by a sense of a hopeful future.

--an increasing balance and integration between the so-called "left" and "right" brains.

The unused capacities of the human mind to experience, to learn, to think, to envision and to create are enormous. Few of us develop more than a small part of our potentials for intellectual competence and creativity, for a more enriched, multi-faceted consciousness. Our "left brain"-dominated education, emphasizing lineal, thinking logic, rationality, analytical, mathematical thinking and problem solving, tends to foster underdevelopment of our "right brain" intuitive, metaphoric, integrating, holistic capacities.

Wholeness-nurturing counseling, therapy and education must move beyond healing our psyches to enable us to enrich our consciousness, strengthen our intellectual muscles, and enhance our sense of psychic aliveness. To love God with all our minds (Mark 12:30) requires life-long holistic learning. With our increased longevity, the people-nurturing institutions of our society--especially our schools and religious institutions--face a demanding challenge to provide a rich variety of learning experiences and networks, so that people may learn how to learn and enjoy the adventures of the mind at each stage of their life journey. Each stage offers new opportunities to expand the horizons of understanding, to cope creatively with the basic issues of living, and to contribute to the needs of the human family.

(3) THE HEALING AND ENLIVENING OF OUR RELATIONSHIPS

The third dimension of our wholeness is the wholeness of our network of significant relationships. In a profound psychological-spiritual sense we humans not only <u>have</u> relationships, we <u>are</u> our relationships. For better or for worse, we are "members of each other" (as the New Testament puts it). The will-to-relate is more fundamental than the will-to-pleasure (Freud), the will to power (Adler), or even the will-to-meaning (Frankl), since only in meaningful relationships can we satisfy any of these essential drives. For human beings, wholeness in all its dimensions is essentially relational. The health of our "caring community" influences profoundly the individual wholeness of everyone within that social system. Growth toward increased body-mind wholeness both feeds and is fed by growth in interpersonal wholeness. The quality of our inner lives and the quality of our intimate relationships enhance or diminish each other reciprocally.

What are some identifying characteristics of relationship wholeness?

Persons are whole in this dimension to the degree that they:

--are themselves growing and are nurturing wholeness in each other.

--communicate clearly, openly and congruently.

--are able to both give and receive love and nurture self-esteem mutually.

--relate in ways that invite creative interdependence and equality with others, not identity-fusing, symbiotic dependency, or hierarchical relationships.

--accept and even appreciate individual differences and autonomy.

--renegotiate changes in their relationship "contract" to keep it just and satisfying to both parties.

Family therapist Virginia Satir points out that growth flourishes in family systems in which the implicit rules are fair, flexible, human and open to renegotiation as the family situation changes and individual members grow. Furthermore, such growthful families are open systems which interact in mutually fulfilling ways with individuals, families and institutions outside the family's boundaries (Satir, 1964, pp. 26-27).

The healing of the alienation in close relationships through direct therapeutic intervention in social systems (e.g., as in conjoint marriage and family therapy) is a valuable development in therapeutic methods. But wholeness-oriented counselors, therapists and teachers, need to go beyond the repair of fragmented relationships, to help people learn the relationship-building skills which will enable them to develop the unused potentials in face-to-face relationships (e.g., the latent marriage in most actual marriages).

In the relational dimension, as in the other dimensions of wholeness, healing approaches and growth approaches complement each other. For example, the therapeutic results of marriage counseling can best be sustained by involving couples in ongoing marriage support groups and enrichment events. Conversely, the awarenesses which are created by effective marriage enrichment programs often help couples who need marriage crisis counseling to recognize their need, come out of hiding, and seek help sooner than would otherwise occur.

To summarize this section, this is the practice-oriented definition of "love" which I find useful in working with wholeness issues in relationships: Love is caring about and commitment to each other's full becoming. The overarching goal of relationship counseling therapy and education is to help people learn how to implement covenants of mutual wholeness.

(4) HEALING AND ENLIVENING OUR INSTITUTIONS

The fourth dimension of wholeness is the wholeness of our interaction with those wider social systems--organizations, institutions, political, economic and religious systems--which sustain or stymie our wholeness. Growth toward greater wholeness in individuals and intimate relationships can flourish fully only in communities whose institutions sustain and nurture wholeness. Unfortunately, many of our culture's institutions are infected with oppressive social malignancies--e.g. sexism, racism, ageism, tribal exclusivism, militarism, nationalism, economic exploitation and political oppression--which cripple human wholeness on a massive scale while we counselors, healers and teachers attempt to heal the crippling of persons on an individual basis. Obviously this is a losing battle. Two-thirds of our sisters and brothers on planet earth face the ravages of hunger, disease, economic exploitation, and overpopulation. In our world the search for privatized wholeness under whatever name is therefore an unethical luxury of the rich. A systemic understanding of wholeness is essential for many reasons, not the least of which is the fact that privatized wholeness is a <u>cul</u> <u>de</u> <u>sac</u>. At the root of all diminished wholeness in individuals are powerful social deterrents to wholeness.

A basic insight of general systems theory, incorporated in the theory of conjoint family therapy, is that the health of intimate social systems tends to enable or limit the growth toward wholeness of all its members. One can extrapolate from this insight to develop methods for gradually transforming larger social systems to make them better environments for supporting physical, psychological, and relational wholeness.

Therapeutic and educational approaches in this fourth dimension should have two goals--to enable individuals to establish and strengthen their relationships with wholeness-supporting institutions, and to empower persons to work with others (using both educational and political methods) to increase the wholeness of the institutions in which they have some influence. What I call the Gandhi-King-Day-Lee principle is a conceptual tool for wholeness-enablers. Mahatma Gandhi, Dorothy Day (of the Catholic Workers Movement), Martin Luther King, Jr., and Tai Jung Lee (leader of the movement for women's and human rights in Korea), in different cultures and religious traditions, each embodied a complementary commitment of personal-spiritual growth on the one hand, and societal transformation on the other.

Sexism is a cultural poison which constricts all dimensions of wholeness in both women and men, in different ways. Consider body wholeness, for example. Women tend to be alienated from their bodies in our culture by being taught to treat their bodies as sex-objects, and to judge (and often reject) them for not measuring up to the superficial, youth-oriented criteria of Hollywood and Madison Avenue. Thus women establish an I-it relationship with their bodies. We males tend to be programmed to experience our bodies as things to be used in the pursuit of "success" or in proving our maleness as measured by superficial macho criteria. Treating ourselves either as "success objects" or as "sex objects" distances us from the richness of our feelings and our senses, and prevents us from loving our bodies as good mother-father to ourselves. Sexist sources of body alienation are reinforced by dualistic theological views which separate spirit from body, and treat the latter as inferior and a source of evil.

In my experience, the institutional-societal dimension of wholeness is the most difficult to keep integrated with the other dimension in doing counseling and therapy. Most of us healers are not trained to think systemically when we work with individuals and intimate relationships. Or are we accustomed to maintaining awareness of the crucial role of power and powerlessness in all psychological and relational healing? Rollo May's distinction between power <u>against</u> others (manipulative, exploitative, competitive power), power <u>for</u> others (nutrient power) and power <u>with</u> others (integrative power) is useful in conceptualizing the political (power) goals of healing and growth work. (May, 1975).

Powerlessness diminishes wholeness; empowering enhances wholeness. When disadvantaged ghetto residents in Chicago got involved in social action to protest economic exploitation and increase economic justice in their community, some of them experienced increased personality health. Their powerlessness and hopelessness were reduced and their self-esteem increased by learning how to mobilize their collective power to exercise more control over their economic well-being. (Seifert and Clinebell, 1969, pp. 19-22). In this example, the interrelationship of liberation and wholeness are evident. These Chicago residents by working together liberated themselves <u>from</u> some of the institutional injustices of their community; they also liberated themselves <u>to</u> greater psychological wholeness.

The common motif which links all the liberation movements of our planet is the insistence that all persons have full and fair opportunities to develop their God-given capacities and potentialities! If we teachers, counselors and healers are to be liberators of this wholeness, empowerment must be a central goal of our work.

(5) HEALING AND ENLIVENING OUR RELATIONSHIP TO THE BIOSPHERE

The fifth dimension of our wholeness is the wholeness of our relationship with the ecosystem. Ecological wholeness involves opening up and deepening our relationship with the natural environment within which we live and which lives in us. Personal wholeness is diminished by our alienation from the great mother of all things living, Mother Nature. We need the re-creation of body, mind, spirit, and relationships which come from opening ourselves to celebrate and enjoy our organic interrelatedness with the natural world. Developing ecological awareness, consciences and caring is essential, for interrupting the rape of nature; it is also essential for our own wholeness. The spiritual heritage of many tribes of Native Americans with their sense of affinity with and respect for nature offers us resources for nurturing ecological wholeness. Of all the dimensions of wholeness, we have had the least practice in facilitating this aspect.

(6) HEALING AND ENLIVENING OUR SPIRITS

The sixth dimension of our wholeness is the wholeness of our spiritual lives, our "higher Selves" (Assagioli, 1971). This dimension, like the axle of a wheel, is the unifying center of the other five. Spiritual wholeness is the heart of all human wholeness because it has to do with those things which most clearly distinguish and define us as human. The degree of our spiritual wholeness is determined by the quality of our values and meanings, our philosophies of life and belief systems, our moments of self-transcendence, and, ultimately, the quality of our relationship with Spirit, the source of all healing and wholeness. Enlivening our relationship with God, the values which guide our choices and determine our life-style, and the meanings which give our lives purpose--all these have profound influences on the wholeness of the other five dimensions. The key of human wholeness is a spiritual key. A growing, nourishing, enlivening relationship with the Spirit of the universe is the source of the energy of growth toward wholeness. I will explore this crucial dimension in more depth below.

THE UNITY OF THE SIX DIMENSIONS

Wholeness involves the organic unity in an integrated, balanced, interaction among these six dimensions. Clinical evidence shows that our wellness is diminished by the splitting of these aspects of our lives, the underdevelopment of some and the overdevelopment of others. The academic structures and professional specialization of Western cultures compartmentalizes these aspects of the whole, dividing concern for them among different academic disciplines, institutions and professions.

It is important to recognize that an individual's potentialities for healing and wholeness are within that person's <u>total</u> situation. All aspects of our lives, our cultural and historical settings, offer limitations and resources for growth. Furthermore, our wholeness options are continually evolving. Each life stage, each change in our personal, historical or cultural situation brings fresh possibilities and new limitations in all of the dimensions and in our lives. In the flow of one's passing years, today's choices expand or limit tomorrow's wholeness possibilities. Thus a person's wholeness potential is a dynamic, developing stream, not a fixed quantity.

On the following page is my favorite right-brain image for depicting these six dimensions of wholeness.

It is noteworthy that the roots of the flower go down deep into the nourishing earth--the ground of our collective being in which we all are profoundly interrelated. The spiritual center of the flower is the place where the seeds of new life grow.

THE FLOWER OF WHOLENESS

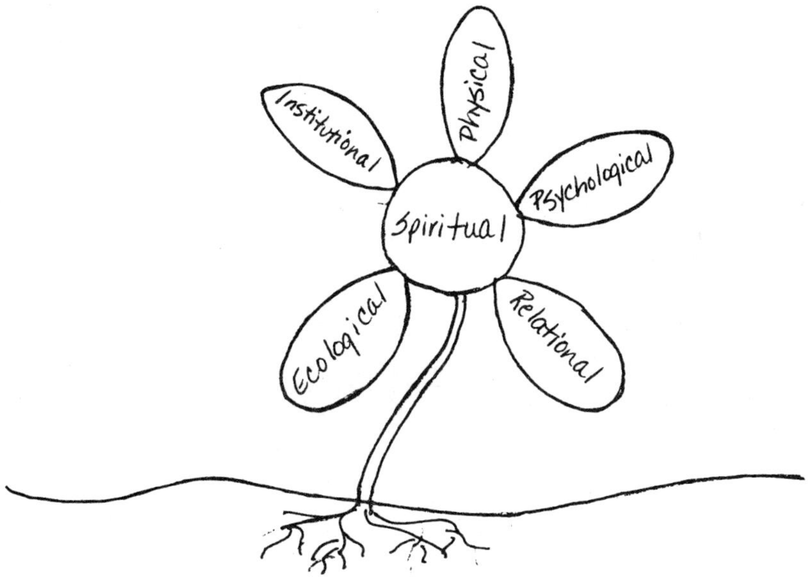

At the first Institute for Religion and Wholeness public meeting in December 1981 (at which I had presented the above image), I was gratified that Nell Morton offered what I regard as a more adequate way of imaging the interrelationship of the six dimensions of wholeness. (Please see figure on next page.) Here is her commentary on this image of wholeness:

> Wholeness is never static--always in ferment and growth. Since we live in a global community and are rapidly emerging into a cosmic mind, would we not think of spirit as that flow of energy that brings us and the five aspects of wholeness into

dynamic relationship with each other--ever in movement, in tension, interactive and interconnected? Interdependent, invisible--yet powerfully present. (Personal communication, 12/81)

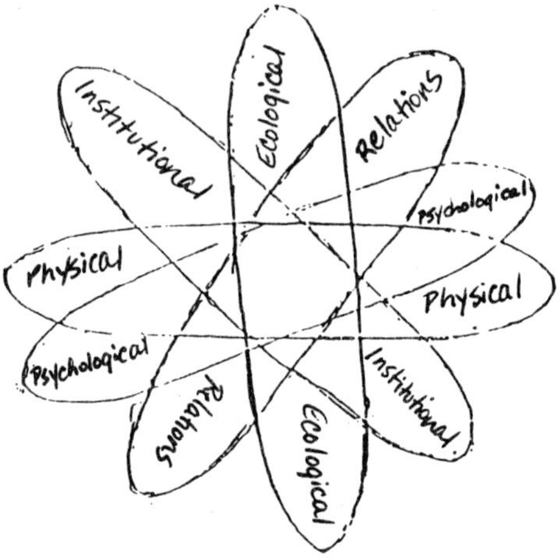

THE NATURE OF THE SPIRITUAL DIMENSION

The spiritual dimension of our lives is the arena in which we seem to satisfy seven interrelated spiritual needs: (1) for a viable philosophy of life; (2) for creative values and ethical sensitivities that serve as constructive guidelines for behavior that is responsible (to the needs of persons) and responsible on both interpersonal and societal levels; (3) for an integrating devotion of a value regarded as ultimate, and a devotion to the divine Spirit which incorporates that value; (4) for developing the higher Self (the "image of God" in the Hebrew Bible) which is the channel through which we experience Spirit in others, in nature, and in direct numinous experience; (5) for a sense of at-homeness, of trustful belonging in the universe; (6) for enlivening "peak experiences" (Maslow), renewing moments of transcendence in which one is open to the Spirit of the universe; (7) for a Spirit-centered, caring community, with shared values and mutual nurturing of spiritual growth (the church or its counterpart).

These needs are human needs, present in all persons, including the most secularized. They are existential in the sense that they are inherent in the nature of human existence. Non-theist Erich Fromm observes: "Because the need for a system of orientation and devotion is an intrinsic part of human existence, we can understand the intensity of this need. There is no other more powerful source of energy in man [sic]" (Fromm, 1950, pp. 25).

More and more people focus their spiritual search for ways to satisfy these needs, outside organized religions. Unless churches and temples become more effective centers for enabling wholeness centered in Spirit, alienation from them will be epidemic.

Our spiritual lives can be crippling or creative, entrapping or liberating of our wholeness. Our religious beliefs and practices can be a <u>weight</u> on our spirit or <u>wings</u> by which we soar! <u>Salugenic</u> (wholeness-enabling) <u>spirituality</u> occurs in the lives of people who satisfy their existential needs in life-affirming, reality-respecting, responsible and growing ways. <u>Pathogenic</u> (sickness-producing) <u>spirituality</u> results when we attempt (always unsuccessfully) to satisfy these needs in rigid, authoritarian, idolatrous, life-constricting, irresponsible and reality-denying ways. The distinction between the "religion of the healthy minded and the sick soul" was described by William James in his classic <u>Varieties of Religious Experience</u>. (Similar distinctions have been articulated by Ruth Benedict, Gordon Allport, Rollo May and others.)

Here are some criteria which can be used in identifying salugenic religion: THE RELIGIOUS BELIEFS, ATTITUDES, AND PRACTICES OF PERSONS ARE WHOLENESS-NURTURING TO THE DEGREE THAT THEY:

--give them a meaningful philosophy of life that provides trust and hope in face of the inevitable tragedies of life.

--provide creative values and ethical sensitivities that serve as inner guidelines for behavior that is both personally and socially responsible.

--provide an integrating, energizing, growing relationship with that loving Spirit that religions call God.

--nurture the transcendent dimensions of persons' lives, their higher Self.

--inspire an ecological love of nature and a reverence for all life.

--provide for a regular renewal of basic trust by affirming a deep sense of belonging in the universe.

--bring the inner enrichment and growth that comes from "peak experiences."

--offer the person a growth-enabling community of caring.

--build bridges rather than barriers between them and persons with differing values and faith systems.

--enhance love and self-acceptance (rather than fear and guilt) in their inner life.

--foster self-esteem and the "owning" of their strengths.

--stimulate the growth of their inner freedom and autonomy.

--help them develop depth relationships commmitted to mutual growth.

--encourage the vital energies of sex and assertiveness to be used in affirmative, responsible ways rather than in repressive or people-damaging ways.

--foster realistic hope by encouraging the acceptance rather than the denial of reality.

--provide them with effective means of moving from the alienation of appropriate guilt to healing reconciliation with themselves, other persons, and God.

--encourage creative change in their beliefs and values to keep these congruent with their intellectual growth.

--provide effective means of keeping in touch with the creative resources of the unconscious through living symbols, meaningful rituals, and vital myths.

--encourage them to keep in touch with both the soft, vulnerable, nurturing, receptive, feelingful side and the assertive, rational, intentional, ethically demanding side of their personalities.

--make them aware of person-hurting institutional practices and motivate them to work to change these forces that oppress potentializing on a massive scale.

--give them the trust, hope, and meaning to face their awareness of death and the inevitable losses of life and to allow their awareness to make living more precious.

--keep them aware of the basic wonder and mystery of all life and growth.

--encourage heightened aliveness and joy and celebration of the good _gift of life_. (Clinebell, 1979, pp. 107-109)

These criteria are stated broadly so they applied to the spiritual dimension of any individual's life, whatever his or her religious background or faith tradition. They can be used diagnostically to identify areas of religious belief or practice in which spiritual healing or growth are needed.

The motivating power of our spiritual needs is derived from two sources. The first is our existential anxiety. We humans are the animals who know we will die. Our nonpathological anxiety regarding death comes from the awesome, often denied awareness that we are all living-dying creatures. Unlike neurotic anxiety, there are no psychological or psychotherapeutic answers to existential anxiety. But the impact of this anxiety can be either deadening and crippling or enlivening and creative, depending on how we respond to it.

Our culture has developed many ways to avoid facing the painful awareness of our mortality. For example, the dynamics of many attempts to escape from existential anxiety by centering life around false absolutes, making a god of work, food, drugs, alcohol, success, family, religion, etc. These are idolatrous attempts to meet profoundly spiritual needs by non-spiritual means. Unfortunately all our psychological idols eventually become demonic.

The other source of the power of our spiritual needs is the fact that we are inherently transpersonal and transcending in our essential natures. Deep within us is the gentle but persistent _élan_ to develop the spiritual core of our being, our higher Self. Both these sources point to the key role of salugenic religion in human wholeness. The only effective way to respond to the awareness of our finitude is to continue to develop wholeness centered in Spirit. The answer to the fear of death is to allow oneself to experience being fully alive in the now, a quality of aliveness which flows from deep spiritual springs. I am beginning to understand the words of a client (years after she uttered them), at the end of her therapy: "When I came for therapy I thought I was afraid of dying, but it turned out I was really afraid of living." Our idolatrous defenses against awareness of our finitude diminish our aliveness and thus render dying all the more threatening.

> The only way to cope creatively with existential anxiety is to risk coming alive now. but this requires existential hope and courage, the courage to be and to become. This courage can come only from an awareness of the ultimate trustworthiness of existence. Salugenic religion is the source of this awareness. By the satisfaction of our deep spiritual hungers, growthful religion provides the existential courage to be and to become, freely and joyfully. (Clinebell, 1979, p. 112)

By experiencing a warm sense of God's love, the "ego chill" (Erik Erikson's term for existential anxiety) is melted and transformed into dynamic motivation to create, to live more fully, to pour one's life energy into the ongoing human journey. If our spiritual experience frees and empowers us to live more fully, death loses its spooky power to frighten us. In the experience of basic trust which comes from Spirit-centered aliveness, existential anxiety is transformed into what Søren Kierkegaard called a "school"--that is, a growth experience empowered by awareness of our finitude.

SPIRITUAL CRISIS AS OPPORTUNITIES

On both personal and societal levels, spiritual crises can be understood and used as occasions for growth toward increased Spirit-centered wholeness. Humankind is caught in a profound spiritual crisis which makes it very difficult to satisfy our spiritual needs growthfully. The awareness of transcendence as an energizing force has largely disappeared from the consciousness of millions of us thing-worshipping people in Western cultures. This has left us in a flat, boring two-dimensional world of materialism with little transcendence or awareness of meaning. The dizzy pace of social change has resulted in a massive breakdown of traditional certainties, beliefs, and value. Authority-centered systems of meaning, and the myths and rituals which expressed and reinforced them, have evaporated like snowballs in hell for countless persons on planet earth. We are in the midst of mind-boggling, spirit-numbing, anxiety-saturated shaking of old religious ways of satisfying spiritual needs and thereby cope with existential anxiety. An epidemic of spiritual pathologies rooted in existential loneliness has been produced by the spiritual vacuum of our time of transition to a new age. Simplistic spiritual solutions from the radical right are proclaimed by religious demagogues who know how to exploit the anxieties of our age for their own self-aggrandizement and wealth. Spiritually impoverished people seek to escape from the new spiritual freedom of our period of history into the comfort of oversimplified "solutions" to the complex spiritual problems of human existence.

When viewed from the wholeness perspective, our planetary spiritual crisis (as well as our personal spiritual crises which proliferate in this context) can be seen as unprecedented opportunities for spiritual growth! The fact that so many of us no longer find the ready-made answers from religious institutions and authority figures believable or personally helpful makes it necessary for us to take responsibility for struggling to find meaningful answers to fundamental ethical and theological issues ourselves. Humankind is challenged (as cultures and as individuals) to develop self-validating, ethical guidelines and belief systems that are relevant to and helpful in living responsibly in the strange new world of the 80's and 90's. The enormous surge of spiritual searching in recent years is hopeful evidence that many people are wrestling with the crucial issues addressed by this conference. A new trans-materialist world view that makes a central place for spiritual reality seems to be emerging from diverse sources including modern physics.

ALCOHOLISM AND THE SIX DIMENSIONS

To relate my theoretical discussion of the six dimensions of wholeness to a particular form of human brokenness, I will now focus on the multiple-faceted sickness called alcoholism. I will seek to show how understanding of both the etiology and the recovery process can be illuminated by viewing this addiction through this theoretical perspective. (I cannot discuss the relation of ecological wholeness to alcoholism because this issue has not yet been explored, to my knowledge.)

There is considerable evidence that physiological and biochemical factors play a significant role in the etiology of alcoholism. These may be the consequences of prolonged excessive drinking rather than predisposing factors. It is probable that there are as yet undetermined physiological factors in the loss of control over one's drinking which is the sine qua non of addiction. There may be irreversible biochemical changes which account for the fact that very few persons who move from controlled to uncontrolled drinking succeed in returning for long to controlled drinking.

Medical treatment often is needed especially in the early stages of recovery. This often includes detoxification procedures and vitamin therapy to help the body repair the nutritional problems resulting from the consumption of most of one's calories in the form of alcohol. Physical rehabilitation of persons suffering from the effects of binges and prolonged excessive drinking frequently increases the likelihood that permanent sobriety will be achieved.

Moving to the second dimension, there are few students of alcohol addiction who believe that there is a unique "pre-alcoholic personality," a distinctive syndrome of psychological attributes which predispose to alcoholism. However, the following attributes have been mentioned repeatedly in reports of psychological studies of alcoholics: high levels of anxiety in interpersonal relationships, emotional immaturity, ambivalence toward authority, low frustration tolerance, narcissism and grandiosity, low self-esteem, feelings of psychological isolation, perfectionism, intense guilt feelings, and compulsiveness. (Clinebell, 1968, p. 53). These attributes probably are present to some degree in many alcoholics before they began drinking uncontrolledly. The increasingly heavy drinking which usually precedes loss of control is motivated in part by the need for alcohol to anesthetize psychological pain. As the addiction develops a self-feeding cycle emerges. The person drinks more excessively to overcome the physical, psychological and interpersonal pain of previous excessive drinking. The more the person drinks, the more he or she needs to drink. Interrupting this addictive cycle is essential if any therapy is to be effective in producing long-term sobriety. Physical detoxification (and sometimes Antabuse), psychological reinforcement (e.g., the AA approach is to help the person learn not to take the first drink), and interpersonal support and modeling of other alcoholics (as in AA or in group therapy) often are instrumental in interrupting the cycle.

Deficiencies in the relationship of wholeness are crucial in understanding both the etiology and treatment of alcoholism. Studies of the dynamics of family systems in which one member is an alcoholic show that alcoholism is a family illness. For example, the marital interaction in such families often exacerbates the problem drinking--e.g., a wife nags, threatens and withholds, and then overprotects the alcoholic, in response to the excessive drinking, which increases his motivation to drink. ALANON's concept of "release" is a way by which the non-alcoholic spouse interrupts her or his side of the neurotic interaction which feeds the addictive cycle.

The key role of relational factors in recovery is illustrated by the effectiveness of the AA sponsor system and the informal group therapy of AA meetings.

The majority of those who achieve sobriety through AA do so without professional therapy. But some alcholics also require counseling, psychotherapy (individual or group) and/or marriage counseling to help heal the underlying psychological and relational problems which otherwise make their sobriety precarious.

To move to the fourth dimension of wholeness, the sanctions, attitudes, and institutionalized needs and customs of various cultures and subcultures play a major role in determining the rates of alcohlism in those cultures. Deeply conflicted and ambivalent attitudes toward drinking and drunkenness in North American culture provide the soil of addiction within which the seeds of addiction (within individuals and family systems) take easy root. A cross-cultural study of some twenty-five cultures revealed that the more a given culture pushes alcohol on people, regards alcohol as an appropriate way of handling stress, and accepts drunkenness as "normal" behavior, the less psychopathology is required for one to become addicted. (Clinebell, 1968, pp. 304-5) The oft-cited example of cultural-institutional variables in alcoholism rates is the contrast between the high incidence among Irish and the very low incidence among orthodox Jews. (As an Irish put it, "You don't have to be Irish to be an alkie, but it helps.") Studies of female alcoholics reveal how the ways in which women are defined and define themselves in a sexist society contribute to the etiology of their addiction. Social desperation drinking among Native Americans and among some other ethnic minorities who suffer painful discrimination and economic exploitation is another example of how cultural variables, like racism, provoke alcoholism.

If one follows the problem of alcoholism to its societal and cultural roots, it opens into a huge mass of intertwined social problems in our tangled civilization. In his comments on the novel The Lost Weekend, Christopher Morley wrote: "It becomes almost the history of the whole era of frustration." (Jackson, 1949, p. 1) It is clear that widespread prevention of problem drinking and alcoholism will depend on basic changes in our society's attitudes and sanctions.

I have explored the philosophical-religious factors in the etiology and treatment of alcoholism elsewhere (Clinebell, 1963). Let me highlight some key points in this area. There is evidence from many sources of connections between excessive drinking and fear of death, value emptiness, religious strivings, meaninglessness and general spiritual malaise. Bill W., co-founder of AA once said: "Before AA we were trying to find God in a bottle." (Personal communication). William James in his Gifford lectures declared, "The sway of alcohol over mankind is unquestionably due to its power to stimulate the mystical faculties of human nature, usually crushed to earth by the cold facts and dry criticisms of the sober hour . . . the drunken consciousness is one bit of the mystical consciousness" (James, 1902, p. 378). In explaining to Big Daddy the great importance of alcohol in his life, Brick, the alcoholic son in Cat on a Hot Tin Roof, says, "A drinking man's someone who wants to forget that he isn't still young and believing." The evidence from cross-cultural anthropology and from the history of religions is also highly suggestive. For example, Dionysus, god of wine, was also related to the afterlife. He was believed to suffer, die and rise from the dead.

Clinical evidence also supports the view that the spiritual component often is crucial in the etiology of and recovery from alcohol addiction. A woman in her early forties came for counseling because of her concern about her rapidly increasing dependence on alcohol. As she discussed her childhood she mentioned a persistent fear of being outside under the stars at night. Closer examination of this and other fears disclosed a common underlying theme--an intense fear of dying, which included both neurotic and existential anxiety. The fear of death has been a common theme among a number of early-stage alcoholics with whom I have counseled. The search for a pseudo-mystical experience through alcohol also occurs frequently among alcoholics at various stages of addiction, as well as among non-alcoholics.

The spiritual problems of alcoholics are not merely derivative from deeper personality problems. They constitute genuine causative factors in their own right. For many alcoholics, alcohol is not just a meaningful symbol of the transcendent dimension of life (as it is in many religious traditions including Christianity). It becomes their _only_ transcendent dimension. As the illness progresses, they tend increasingly to seek satisfaction of all their spiritual needs through alcohol. Alcohol become the _summum bonum_ for them pushing out all other values.

For the alcoholic, alcohol eventually proves to be a Janus-faced god. Its hidden face is the face of a devil who betrays the alcoholic's trust in it. It may be that it is when alcohol loses its pseudo-religious power--its power to bring temporary unity, meaning, transcendence and closeness to others--that the alcoholic "hits bottom" and becomes open to help.

It is no accident that the most effective treatment program ever devised in the long dark history of alcoholism--AA--is essentially a spiritual program (derived from the Oxford Group Movement). The 12 suggested Steps of recovery emphasize turning one's life over to a higher power--God as one understands him. These steps encourage positive surrender to the higher Power, dealing with the enormous load of alienation and guilt (through the moral inventory), cultivating a conscious contact with God through prayer and meditation, and reaching out to other alcoholics to share one's experience of transformation. A "spiritual awakening" is expected to result from this process.

In 1961, Bill W. wrote to Carl Jung to thank him for being instrumental in helping his friend Roland to sobriety. In his letter of response Jung expressed the view that the alcoholic's craving for alcohol is a "spiritual thirst for wholeness" and that the spiritual experience which is [often] necessary for sobriety, occurs when one walks a path leading to a higher understanding." (AA Grapevine, January, 1963). Several years ago it dawned on me that I had never known (in three decades of interest in alcohol addiction) an alcoholic who had achieved long-term, stable sobriety without having experienced significant growth toward Spirit-centered wholeness.

References

Assagioli, A., Psychosynthesis, A Manual of Principles and Techniques. New York: Viking, 1971.

Clinebell, H., Contemporary Growth Therapies. Nashville: Abingdon Press, 1981.

Clinebell, H., Growth Counseling, Hope-Centered Methods of Actualizing Human Wholeness. Nashville: Abingdon Press, 1979.

Clinebell, H., Philosophysical-Religious Factors in the Etiology and Treatment of Alcoholism. Quarterly Journal of Studies on Alcohol, Sept., 1962.

Clinebell, H., Understanding and Counseling the Alcoholic. Nashville: Abingdon Press, 1968.

Fromm, E., Psychoanalysis and Religion. New Haven: Yale University Press, 1950.

Jackson, D., The Lost Weekend. New York: New American Library, 1948.

James, W., Varieties of Religious Experience: A Study in Human Nature. New York: Longman, Green, 1902.

Keen, S., To a Dancing God. New York: Harper and Row, 1970.

Lowen, A., The Betrayal of the Body. New York: Collier Macmillan, 1967.

Lowen, A., Sexuality, Sex and the Human Potential, Human Potentialities, H. Otto (Ed.), St. Louis: Warren H. Green, 1968.

May, R., Power and Innocence. New York: Wiley, 1975.

Maslow, A., Toward a New Psychology of Being. New York: Van Nostrand, 1968.

Satir, V., Peoplemaking. Palo Alto, CA: Science and Behavior Books, 1964.

Seifert, H. and Clinebell, H., Personal Growth and Social Change. Philadelphia: Westminster Press, 1969.

ECOLOGICAL OR ENVIRONMENTAL WHOLENESS

Religion and Wholeness in the Shadow of Modernity

D.S. Pacini

> . . . Origin makes possible a field of knowledge whose function is to recover it, but always in a false recognition due to the excesses of its own speech.
>
> --Foucault

How are we to speak of religion and wholeness, or can we speak of it at all? This query, put with increasing and suspicious frequency in centers of religious study, questions the very credentials of the subject: it suggests that the link between religion and wholeness, however it may have been conceived in the past, is today dead or dying. The principal symptoms that seem to support this belief are the absence of any commanding works on the subject in the twentieth century and the growing influence of Nietzsche on late twentieth-century religious thought, especially through the work of Heidegger, Foucault, Derrida, Altizer, Raschke, Taylor, Windquist, and Scharlemann, the effect of which appears to be to reduce still further the likelihood that questions of this variety will have any standing at all.

This, of course, is scarcely conclusive evidence. It may be that central presuppositions of this question are no longer acceptable, because they, together with the world of which they were a part, have withered away or become discredited. Or it may also be that new disciplines have taken over the work of older ways of thinking that today we view as instances of systematic delusions; we regard alchemy and astrology in this way, as do many of our critics theology and metaphysics. In any event, these possibilities, if real, would certainly signal the demise of the question of religion and wholeness and the ways of thinking that attend it.

Even so, it would be mistaken to presume that having shuffled this question into one or another of these well-organized compartments we will have resolved what confusions of thought surround the issue of religion and wholeness. For we have yet to divest the issue of the distortions of thought that have accrued to it and that we have appropriated uncritically. One of the distortions is that it is possible to formulate the issue of religion and wholeness apart from historical considerations; with one foot, however reluctantly, still sunk in historical soil, advocates of this view show signs of a tendency to tear themselves loose and emancipate themselves from the main body in which they were born, much as proponents of the modern sciences did in their day. The purpose of this essay is to indicate that this line of thought, illuminating as it may be in various unintended ways, rests upon a fallacy that still obsesses the thought of many distinguished contemporary religious thinkers.

I

Nietzsche wrote of his most trusted friend, Franz Overbeck, in late November 1880:

> I want nothing more to do with the concerns of contemporary "idealism," especially the German variety. Let's all do our own work, posterity

> will set us in proper order anyhow, or maybe it won't.[1]

He wrote Overbeck again in June of 1881:

> As far as Christianity is concerned, I hope you'll believe this much: in my heart I've never held it in contempt, and, ever since childhood, have often struggled with myself on behalf of its ideals. In the end, to be sure, the result has always been the sheerest impossibility . . .[2]

Nietzsche's letters were prompted in part by the completion and publication of The Dawn of Day and the development of themes for his newest project, The Gay Science. The deceit of history had become a central preoccupation of Nietzsche's puzzling. In The Dawn of Day, he noted that the anti-Enlightenment revisionist conception of history as the sympathetic study of the origin, and development of the past had become the vehicle for the reassertion of the Enlightenment outlook on scientific history.[3] In his celebrated apostrophe against history, "Historiabscondita," which appeared in The Gay Science, Nietzsche quipped that every great human being becomes a source of illumination by which the secrets of the past are brought into view, thereby precipitating the sense that "there is no way of telling what may yet become history some day."[4] Nietzsche's criticisms were anchored in the suspicion that most forms of historical inquiry either introduce or presuppose a supra-historical perspective. On the one hand scientific history, characteristic of the resurgent Enlightenment, was persuaded that the field of our lives is an inexorably fixed time order. Some natural law governs the order and shaping of events that affect human lives and activities, and this law can be known through the patterns of events that disclose regularities. Moreover, it becomes plausible to conceive of the regular succession of events in terms of cause and effect. Such laws, of course, are eternal and unchangeable, equally applicable in all times and all places. But they are, as well, suprahistorical, and the history that depends upon them is based upon a standpoint that is outside of time.

On the other hand, those who subscribed to the revisionist conception of history held that its distinctive methods and canons, no less exacting, perhaps, than those of the sciences of nature, rested on foundations different from them. The subjective, impressionist embodiment of personal vision that would reduce the diversity of time into a totality fully reconciled with itself was hardly less rigorous a conception of history. Yet it, too, bases itself in a perspective outside of time, according privileged position to apocalyptic objectivity.

These modes of historical thinking of which Nietzsche counterpoised his own reflections were not, of course, exhaustive. Others held that the subjective character of history precluded the possibility of systemic rigor, or, what amounted to a variation of this, that its subjective character lent itself to the category of art. But in the main, the modes of historical thinking that worried Nietzsche were the Enlightenment and revisionist conceptions of history, and these, it must be added, were indissolubly linked with the dominant ways in which religion was conceived. Once this linkage is brought into view, it becomes clear that what Nietzsche opposed in religious theories was their unreal, thin, and even absurd assumptions about the nature of social development.

What were these religious views? There was, of course, the Kantian view that carefully circumscribed the bounds of religion in order to avoid the pitfalls of scepticism and fanaticism. Against the backdrop of the French Enlightenment outlook that construed the race as both subjects and objects of objectifying scientific analysis, Kant offered an ameliorating position. He at once sustained the canons of scientific thought and established a distinct realm of moral and religious belief and conduct. What Kant meant by this has been widely debated, but this much seems clear: the canons appropriate to scientific thinking are no more than "analogously" applicable to the moral and religious sphere. However much Kant wanted to assert the primacy and reality of moral feeling, and to underscore the assurance that good deeds would issue (ultimately) in good results, he could not depart from the normative status of scientific, instrumental thinking. For this reason, Kant's notion that moral religion consists in the heart's disposition to fulfill all human duties as divine commands lacked sufficient motivating power;[5] by observing the limits of scientific knowledge, the assertion of God's existence can never extend to a description of God's being, but can only be made as an assumption for the sake of our ethical lives. It was unclear, therefore, that the motivation for moral acts did not in some sense still derive from contingent desires subject to the Newtonian skein of cause and effect.

A prominent advocate of Christian orthodoxy, Gottlob Christian Storr, seized upon this defect, and argued, in effect, that the only sufficient motivating power for rational morality is religious convictions whose credibility can be derived from historical criticism of sacred text. Storr's position contributed to the other view of religion, which, for purposes of inclusivity, I shall refer to as "expressionism," following the suggestion of Isaiah Berlin.[6] It seemed to Storr's radical young students at Tübingen Seminary that his teaching was a perversion of the intentions of Kant. Because there appeared to be justification for Storr's position in some of Kant's theoretical writings, the young seminarians became convinced that in order to preserve the proper spirit of Kant, the letter of his teachings had to be changed. The views of Johann Georg Hamann, Friedrich Heinrich Jacobi, and Johann Gottfried Herder commanded the attention of this group, largely because they ran counter to those aspects of Kant's theories that were still anchored in the thought of the French Enlightenment. Paradoxically, these Counter-Enlightenment views re-introduced the rocks of scepticism and mysticism (fanaticism) Kant had tried to avoid and upon which he thought his argument would not come to wreck.

Hamann and Jacobi had indeed derived much of their anti-rationalist outlook from David Hume's attack upon the possibility of an a priori route to reality, although they turned his views to altogether different ends.[7] Whereas Hume's scepticism sought to discredit religious mysticism, Hamann's and Jacobi's was deployed to defend it. For Hamann, systems of thought are prisons of the spirit. Rationalism, in particular, is a vast distortion of reality. What matters is not concepts, theories, or systems, but insight that springs from feeling. The inner personal life of the individual, art, personal relationships, and religious experience, are the sources of true knowledge. The particular and the concrete are always real: no theory can adequately recapitulate the reality of a gesture, a look, a tone. To understand, accordingly, is to grasp the qualities that shape experience, and this is possible only from the standpoint of naive, intimate trust.[8]

Hamann's disciple, Jacobi, continued this line of thought. Faith, according to Jacobi, is the one genuine form of knowledge. Our certainty of our own existence and of our own unique personality is a sense of reality that is not susceptible to rational deduction. Yet this sense of reality guarantees the reality of whatever is revealed to us. It follows from this that faith or the fundamental sense of reality is the touchstone of all knowledge; because we believe in our senses, we believe as well in the reality of the sensible world. Cogent, rational systems of logical, mathematical, or metaphysical constructions are no more than castles in the air.[9]

Herder was another of Hamann's disciples. Following his teacher, Herder maintained that to understand anything required understanding it in its individuality and development. Such understanding entails empathy with the unique character of the artistic traditions, literature, social organizations and culture of people. Individuals are not the atomistic concatenation of the Enlightenment view, but instead are expressive beings. Through such expression the unity that constitutes the essence of human life comes into view, and with it the awareness that human life is embedded in, and not opposed to, nature. Religion, accordingly, is the expression of traditions, created by entire societies living in an integrated communal life. It is one of the indissoluble and impalpable ties by which persons are joined to communities; indeed, it is the bearer of a certain culture that is sustaining for its members.[10]

Schelling, Hegel, and Holderlin appropriated and developed these teachings in different ways, but in their earliest writings, it is clear that the conception of the expressive dimension of human beings afforded them a way to speak of religion that did not succumb to the excessive formalism of Kant and the austere orthodoxy of Storr. Under the influence of their mentor, Johann Gottlieb Fichte, Schelling and Holderlin learned to criticize Kant's assumption that the ultimate principle of mind and nature is formal unity. Fichte claimed that the ultimate principle is opposition, a force of action beyond the individual and in terms of which our consciousness and its moral law are to be understood.[11] Schelling pursued this line of argumentation, attempting to unite Spinoza with Fichte. Just as Spinoza had argued that Deus sive natura, Schelling now claimed that the all is in the absolute ego, and the "absolute ego is nothing but God."[12] Religion, as the belief in God, is the return of finite consciousness to its absolute origin. Holderlin, somewhat more circumspect than Schelling, accepted the centrality of opposition, but conceived of it as derivative, as the consequence of judgement; accordingly, knowledge and action aim properly to restore the original unity, which is love.[13] In this way, Holderlin hoped to guarantee the freedom of feeling, and beauty of life in thought.

Cognizant of these developments, the young Hegel began to sketch out ways to protect the true spontaneity of life from the compulsive systems of institutions, especially the asceticism of the church. His interest soon turned to theoretical sketches showing how this spontaneity could liberate itself from the subjection of an utterly alien set of circumstances and again express itself as the religious essence of human beings.[14]

Hegel, Schelling, and Holderlin were not the only circle of friends developing the expressionist view of religion. In a different circle, yet under kindred influences, Novalis, Tieck, Friedrich Schlegel, Wachenroder, and Schleiermacher entertained different approaches to the interpretation of religion that would extricate it both from the distortions of the Enlightenment outlook and the severity of extreme Kantian moralism. For this group, the appeal of Spinoza, mediated by Jacobi, and of the theoretical speculations of Fichte was especially powerful; Goethe, too, loomed powerfully in their discussions.

None of the views to emerge from these discussions is more famous, perhaps, than those of the young Schleiermacher pressed relentlessly to prove that their formulations were inept. Religion, he held, is no more to be found in the domain of ethics and aesthetics than it is to be derived from the speculations of physics and metaphysics. Rather, religion is a sense and taste of the infinite that is prior to and imbues our various ways of knowing and doing.[15] So understood, religion is an affection, a kind of pre-reflective awareness, by which the infinite reveals itself in the finite. Insofar as Schleiermacher conceives of the infinite as the whole, religion cannot be comprehended under any single form, but only under the sum total of all forms. Thus religion rescues us from narrow-mindedness and one-sidedness from the fetters of dogma, opinion, and selfish desire.

In his more mature writings, Schleiermacher came to focus upon the mediating role of the historical traditions of which we are a part. Consistent with his earlier views, Schleiermacher claims that we could not form adequate conceptualization of the pre-reflective awareness, but went on to say that our appropriation of this sense is shaped by the communities of our lives. To speak of religion, accordingly, is both to acknowledge a pre-reflective commonality that we intimate and to delineate the specific traditions through which it is communicated.

Given these broad outlines of both the Kantian and expressionist views of religion, it is not difficult to discern their fundamental affinities with the Enlightenment and Counter-Enlightenment or revisionist conceptions of history. The Kantian view of religion and the Enlightenment conception of history hold in common the assumption that there is one set of universal and unalterable principles that govern the affairs of the race. So, too, human nature is fundamentally the same in all times and places, consisting, as it were, of a constant central core, in terms of which universal goals could be derived and verified through a logically connected structure of scientific laws. The Expressionist conception of religion and Counter-Enlightenment conception of history rejected scientific universality, objectivity, rationality, and the belief in the human capacity to provide permanent solutions to all genuine problems of thought. In place of the Enlightenment belief in applying rational and scientific methods to the organization of life, there arose the commitment to the internal human world of morality, art, language, forms of expression, thought and feeling. The products of human creation--music, law, poetry, mathematics--although imbued with the effects of the finite encounter with the Infinite, are nonetheless thoroughly intelligible, because they are the products of the human mind.

When viewed together in just this way, the Enlightenment conception of history and the Kantian view of religion exhibit common beliefs about social development, just as do the Counter-Enlightenment conception of history and the expressionist view of religion. Social development, they thought, was a matter of human progression that depends upon unquestioning faith in the main features of a framework that weaves the threads of political, social, economic, and religious institutions into the fabric of the languages, ideals, modes of feeling, and habits that function to promote the welfare of a people. Where the Enlightenment-Kantian view differed from the Counter-Enlightenment-Expressionist view, of course, was in its assessment of what characteristics made such a framework adequate. But disputes over scientific law or some variant of natural law, even in its highly individualized hybrid form, scarcely veiled their deeper shared conviction that there is some metaphysic, some eternal truth, that discloses the form of history and of social development in a lasting and influential way.

It is hardly surprising that Nietzsche found these views equally abhorrent. Placing, as they do, everything considered eternal within a process of historical development, such views impart to historical understanding the ill-conceived notion that history is a manifestation of continuity. To Nietzsche's way of thinking, the notion of continuity suppresses the irregularities of experience "that give color to it," and overlooks "the consequences for a regular arrangement of work" that flow from "the different ways of dividing the day."[16] For this reason, Nietzsche propounded the view that traditional devices for constructing a comprehensive view of history and for retracing the past in a patient and continuous development had to be dismantled. History, he claims, introduces discontinuities into our being, "the iron hand of necessity shaking the dice box of chance."[17] History discloses the profusion of entangled events which disrupt our sense that our world is a simple configuration of events exemplifying meaning and value.

Whenever a thinker, no matter how distant from us in time or culture, evokes a passionate response within us, be it of enthusiasm or of indignation, it is quite probably the case that the general line of thought advanced pertains to some deeply established conventional wisdom. This is as true of Nietzsche as it is of his current disciples, who have set out to recast Nietzsche's preoccupations for the contemporary scene. Organizing religious thought from Kant to Lotze, Durkheim, and Troeltsch, or from Schleiermacher, Weber, and Otto along the familiar lines of the Enlightenment Christian tradition or of the Counter-Enlightenment expressionist tradition is almost a conviction with us, and having that disturbed causes us acute discomfort.

Paradoxical as it may seem, Nietzsche's way of framing the issues reinforces our conviction that the categories of Enlightenment-Kantian and of Counter-Enlightenment-Expressionism aptly depict the religious and social self-understanding of the age, even if Nietzsche, seeing such self-understanding confining and claustrophobic, demanded more space light. Negating this self-understanding is an exercise in diagnosis whose findings we accept. Where we are likely to depart from Nietzsche is in his prescriptive use of negation to extirpate, to reshape, and to sublimate our desire to believe that the content rests upon profound intentions and immutable necessities. We have been profoundly uneasy with Nietzsche's observation that

> . . . the physicians are still lacking, above all for whom/what we have hitherto called practical morality must be transformed into a piece of their art and science of therapy . . .as yet the churches are not in the hands of the promoters of health . . .[18]

We prefer instead to think of ourselves as makers and doers whose culture runs counter to the principal lines of thought Nietzsche opposed.

Posing with Nietzsche's diagnosis, despite contempt for his prescriptive measure, is more wrong-headed than we have been likely to suppose. For Nietzsche's gaze did not extend beyond the parochial boundaries of a select group of thinkers. His sense of the struggle between the regions of exteriority and inferiority was deeply shaped by these thinkers and their categories, as was his solution. To conceive of Nietzsche's diagnosis as a reading of the self-understanding of the age rather than of a specific culture is a distortion. It reinforces the view that religious nationalism and the metaphysics that supported it are an essential, if not always stated, theme of the period. Those who join Nietzsche in illumining the metaphysics that supported religious nationalism, but who confound them with the metaphysics of the religious outlook of the period do no more than light what Kant called "the magic lantern of phantasms." They fail, as did Nietzsche, to bring into view the religious outlook of the culture that transcended national boundaries and proved to be decisive for the period.

II

Humans fashion their civil world--their civilization and its institutions--not out of whole cloth nor out of infinitely malleable material, but from the ideas, events, and forces that erupt and appear in specific configurations that articulate the experiences of the time. The religious outlook of modernity did not, as has often been supposed, belong to any particular people, but was expressive of a deeper transnational culture. Its voice was to be heard in the emancipatory teachings of what we now call modern physics, modern political and social theory, modern ethics and metaphysics, modern history and international jurisprudence, modern economics and modern philosophy of religion. The initial proponents of this religious outlook were to be found in England, France, Switzerland, Italy, and Holland, all regions of religious intolerance and bitter ecclesiastical, political disputes. Others in Germany, Scandinavia, the United States, Austria, and Russia would soon contribute to the making of this outlook. The most prominent names associated with the foregoing of this view are Grotius, Hobbes, Descartes, Newton, Spinoza, Locke, Rousseau, Smith and Vico. Kant, Hegel, Coleridge, Emerson, Darwin, Marx, and Freud would, in their own ways, develop the possibilities latent within this framework.

What was this view? In brief, it was that all individual entities exhibit certain features--a basic force or capacity and a principle to govern or direct it, together with a reflexive awareness that can thematize the relationship among these components. Locke, perhaps more than anyone else, laid these components bare in his essays on Understanding and on Government, employing the notion of self-preservation as the framework through which these components could be identified.[19] In this paradigmatic use of self-preservation, Locke joined his contemporaries who were setting down the main lines of the modern disciplines.

The idea they had in common was that self-preservation exemplified the emancipatory aspirations of the age. As a reflexive notion, it captured the inward turn away from external authorities, whether ecclesiastical or civil. Grotius, Descartes, Spinoza and Rousseau knew well the sting of ecclesiastical censure, as well as the experience of civil punitive measures. Hobbes, too, knew the requirements of political flight. But more than the exodus from the pressures of social institutions, the idea of self-preservation represented a departure from the outlook of Calvinist and Aristotelian humanism, which subscribed to the belief in pre-ordained goals for all individuals. Despite the relentless efforts of humanism to soften the rigid structures of Orthodoxy through appeals to its sources, Calvinism and Thomism alike grew steadily as the legitimating ideologies for religious intolerance, bigotry, and oppression. The idea, therefore, that there are no pre-ordained goals, no pre-established course that individuals are required to traverse, and no external cause in terms of which the motion of life is to be defined, freed individual reason to choose continuously its own new goals through which the notion of life could be expressed. In self-preservation, one is free to choose; however much Calvinist and Thomist humanists strove to secure free choice, the conceptual framework within which they operated seemed to work at cross-purposes with ther point, no matter how saliently put.

But more than freedom of choice, self-preservation underscored the obligation of choice: in order to preserve oneself, one has to be aware of what one is. Such awareness, however, is impossible apart from the preservation of one's essence. In choosing one form of life, one gives up another, and the great peril, naturally, is that one will choose what is alien to one's essence, thereby initiating self-destruction. It follows from this that there must be some single principle that not only regulates life, but also prescribes the behavior appropriate to all living creatures. A variant of natural law tradition, this principle was unique in that it was thought to reside in the dynamic structure of self-preservation.

It seemed natural enough to define this principle of self-preservation in terms of the individual. Hobbes, Locke, Newton, Descartes, and Spinoza pressed the notion in this way, as did Grotius and Smith. But Grotius and Smith were equally persuaded that this principle undergirded as well a notion of sociability that offset the austere egoism into which individuals could fall. The problem, of course, was how to move from the standpoint of the individual and its principle of survival to the standpoint of society.

Against this there arose the convictions of Vico and Rousseau who conceived of self-preservation as a function of the social organism. Not individual but communities were the basic unit in terms of which self-preservation had to be conceived. Whether through historical understanding that enters imaginatively into the creative endeavors of other peoples in their own terms (Vico) or through moral feeling that intimates the common God (Rousseau), the principle that rightly regulates life could not be discerned apart from interaction with others.

The differences in outlook between the individual and social conceptions of self-preservation cannot be attributed solely to differences in circumstance in the lives of their authors. They derive as well from the unstable structure, the inherent dynamic tension, of the notion of self-preservation. Conceived as the interplay between force and governing principle, the notion of self-preservation lent itself to differing emphases: to depart from the notion of force inevitably committed reflection to the problem of inferiority and individuality, and to conceive of the principle in these terms; whereas to begin with the notion of governing principle commended the view of the social, the interpersonal, the exteriority and to construing the basic force in these terms. Rousseau was something of an exception to this, insofar as he came to recognize that neither individuality nor sociability could be wholly separated from one another. Indeed, for Rousseau, it became clear that force and principle are dialectically related. The expression of the essential force of individual entities is simultaneously the expression of itself or governing principle. For this reason, the individual, in expressing its essence, discovers its true interpersonal character.

It was with Rousseau, as well, that the religious character of this outlook came into view. His contemporaries,. from Grotius to Locke, had understood themselves to have begun with a concept of nature from which they derived the goal of self-knowing virtue. Rousseau, however inadvertently, saw through their arguments to the actual foundation upon which they, collectively understood, rested. The move from the individual standpoint to the social standpoint, which they all professed, could not be successful apart from some means of overcoming the scepticism to which his contemporaries were disposed. Some assurance that those who do good are not deceived, and are therefore fools, is the only impediment to the triumph of wickedness. The promptings of the heart, of conscience, are the expression of the God within and the warrant of such assurances.[20]

Rousseau's unwavering belief in the unbroken human being and of the divine instinct that expresses itself through conscience, his impassioned pleas for direct vision and natural feeling, and his denunciation of the artificial social roles civilization forces the race to play against its true ends, appealed to Hamann and Kant alike, and so to formative figures of what have ordinarily been reckoned competing traditions. Closer in outlook than most have imagined, Kant and Hamann, and those who followed them, differed more in their assessment of Rousseau's timeless truths. Despite everything, Rousseau still believed in the accessibility to these universal principles, for they were indelibly engraved on the hearts of the race. To Hamann and his followers, such precepts were deadly, but to Kant and his successors, they opened the prospect for a theoretical grounding, altogether missing in Rousseau, for the experience of freedom.

This conception of religion, bearing distinct affinities with, and being in some measure derivative of, the Augustinian conception of religion, marked the modern age. As in Augustine's view, the moderns held that something of the original unity of the world (God) can be discovered in each individual through introspection that presses beyond the pretentions of individuality to the restorative power of community.

The various ways in which it was developed notwithstanding, its character remained hidden, even to the astute of the age, owing largely to the failure to resolve the visible dispute between the Enlightenment and Counter-Enlightenment conceptions of history.

III

Although Nietzsche never grasped the actual character of the religious outlook of that age, he nonetheless understood the preoccupation with self-preservation as a paradigm for thought. In The Gay Science, he challenged the fundamental assumption of this doctrine that he largely associated with English thought: "What is called good preserves the species, while what is called evil is harmful to the species."[21] Nietzsche went on to say:

> In truth, however, the evil urges are expedient and indispensible, and preserve the species to as high a degree as the good ones -- only their function is different.22

Nietzsche was not lionizing evil here, however, but quarreling with the presumption that goodness is the energy of the strong or the reaction of the weak. Self-preservation is the eruption of forces into a specific consolidation that is unintelligible apart from the welter of experience. Possibilities, limits, tonalities, and simplicity of form attach themselves to this consolidation. As a specific event, however, and precisely in terms of its specificity, it is utterly marked off from the eternal play of forces. From the perspective of the free play of force, the specific consolidation is the stage upon which the forces meet in threatening confrontation. The relationships played out upon the stage are no more than a scene: they are not eternal verities displayed for all to see.

So understood, self-preservation is a single drama. What Nietzsche did not see was that in its modern dress, self-preservation achieved the form of a religious outlook, whose proponents had seized the rules of the preceding dominating class (the Church), inverted them, and redirected them against those who had initially imposed them. Far from being a successive configuration, the modern religious outlook was a displacement, a disguise and systematic reversal. Only when one sees that modernity was the surreptitious appropriation of a system of rules does its religious outlook come into view.

The identification of the penchant of both the Enlightenment-Kantian view and the Counter-Enlightenment-Expressionist view to dissolve the singular event into an ideal continuity is Nietzsche's achievement. His supposition that religion was encompassed by these traditions was extravagant; to herald the end of the Christian religion, even if, as he conceded, it was beyond the comprehension of many, may have been an error. But he did uncover a mode of historical understanding, something entailed in the notion of reading words, persons, cultures, the past.

No theory of religion and wholeness that resists superficial interpretation, hasty criticism, and the refusal to deal with the distortions and anguish of modern consciousness can afford to turn away from Nietzsche's insight. To develop the insight beyond the confines of the traditional categories that Nietzsche framed for viewing modern religion--categories to which we are predisposed and which commit us to the underlying assumptions with which Nietzsche framed for viewing modern religion--categories to which we are predisposed and which commit us to the underlying assumptions with which Nietzsche rightly quarreled--is the task at hand. The view of religion and social development as a specific, concrete consolidation of the eruption of forces whose metaphysic, if similarity even-specific, may open a path that is sufficient to reveal the tensions we experience but do not understand. Historical thinking that deprives us of the reassuring stability of life and nature, and that disrupts its pretended continuity, affirms the responsibility of thought to make explicit its perspective and to acknowledge its system of injustice.

Footnotes

[1] Nietzsche, Correspondence, ed. Peter Fuss and Henry Shapiro.

[2] Ibid.

[3] The Dawn, 197.

[4] The Gay Science.

[5] Kant, Religion Within the Limits of Reason Alone, IV.

[6] Isaiah Berlin, "Herder and the Enlightenment," Aspects of the Eighteenth Century, ed. Earl Wasserman.

[7] See, for example, Jacobi, David Hume on Belief, 1787.

[8] Hamann, Samtliche Werke, Vol. III.

[9] Jacobi, David Hume on Belief.

[10] Herder, God, Some Conversations.

[11] Fichte, Science of Knowledge, 1794.

[12] Schelling, Correspondence, Samliche Werke.

[13] Holderlin, "Being and Judgment."

[14] Hegel, Early Theological Writings.

[15] Schleiermacher, On Religion: Speeches to the Cultured Among its Despisers.

[16] The Gay Science, 7.

[17] The Dawn, 130.

[18] Ibid., 202.

[19] Locke, Essay Concerning Human Understanding and Two Treaties on Government.

[20] Rousseau, Emile, "Creed of a Priest of Savoy."

[21] The Gay Science, 4.

Wholeness and the King's Men

Catherine Keller

Humpty Dumpty sat on a wall
Humpty Dumpty had a great fall
All the king's horses and all the king's men
Couldn't put Humpty together again.

-- Anonymous

This is what I am: watching the spider
rebuild -- "patiently," they say

but I recognize in her
impatience--my own--

the passion to make and make again
where such unmaking reigns

-- Adrienne Rich

If "such unmaking reigns," it should not come as a surprise that the reigning king's men could not make the broken egg whole again.

Willy-nilly the language of "wholeness" brings with it a world of associations to the female, the feminine, or woman herself: the wholeness of egg, of womb, of contained waters and moonlit web, of undivided or reconciled opposites, of the bond of infant to mother or lover to lover, of an unalienated holiness, a healing, holding inclusion rather than a divisive, exclusive sanctimony, of harmonies rather than hierarchies, of the nervous soothing desire evoked by the image of woman in a culture of unmaking. Therefore it is not only appropriate, it is vital, if we are to avoid the nostalgia that merely sustains a status quo of unwholesome schisms, to hear from women. To hear from women means to listen, without embarrassment or chivalry, to the passions of feminism. For without the feminist impatience, "the Feminine" remains a pastiche of projections promising wholeness and in fact preventing that very passion by which the breakage might be stopped. Therefore I will want to address, from a transparently feminist perspective, the very notion of "wholeness." This transparency is meant to determine not only method, but content, for it is my conviction that feminism itself is more than self-referential, more than a matter of woman's issues, but a window on the dream-broken soul of culture. It affords a privileged view of basic structures of self and relation.

It is quite plausible to describe the journey of women at the end of this millennium as a journey toward wholeness--depending, of course, on the spirit centering it. Wholeness, like that of Humpty Dumpty, is known through its brokenness. The term has no meaning apart from its reference to a presupposed break. This is true now of the term "woman" as well. Woman's fragmentation from other women and from herself has been hidden in the wholesome images of her small sphere of relationships, of her Mona Lisa silence, of her bovine holiness. Only recently has the awareness of the fragmentation brought woman's state to such visibility that it begins to achieve transparency. This hope depends for its wider psychosocial actualization upon the growing awareness on the part of males that as the part contains the whole, the fragments of broken women finally consume, subsume, the dominant man. His wholeness is impossible apart from hers. Thus the universal oppressiveness of the social structures of patriarchy may shed invaluable light on the myriad dichotomies and diseases of our civilization. This hope for wholeness depends, in other words, upon a metapatriarchal therapeutic generated in that fine interplay of the personal and the political, the micro- and macrocosmic. Such a therapeutic is at once radically feminist and a rehearsal for the entire spectrum of holisms: ecological, economic, intercultural, parapsychological, interdisciplinary and just plain interpersonal. For it will recognize the radical connection between all forms of brokenness, and the breakage practiced in the intimately political spheres where sexual caste is brewed.

That wholeness, or something like it, remains a feminist concern that finds testimony in the poem of Adrienne Rich which seems to answer, by its parallelism of web-imagery, the "impatience" of "Natural Resources" (above). It is called "Integrity," and its epigraph quotes Webster's definition: "the quality or state of being complete; unbroken condition; entirety." We should note that the word "integrity" has a different set of connotations than "wholeness," though the denotation is well-nigh identical. Integrity suggests a moral or ethical rightness, wholeness a soundness of health. Further, integrity, with its mathematical association to "integer" and its suggestion of an activity of integration presupposing differentiation, evokes the composition of the whole out of other wholes, more an action perhaps than a state, a way of being rather than an ideal. I am not proposing one term over another, only pointing at distinctions.

The poem opens in direct response to her earlier stage of self: "A wild patience has taken me this far." The psychological distance thus measured is described in this epiphany, like the ego eimi of the Johannine Jesus without the tone of arrogant certainty: "Nothing but myself? . . . My selves." After so long, this answer. "This pluralism of selfhood seems to me a vital clue in the formulation of feminist criteria of wholeness, or integrity. But the dimension underlying the search for clues, and requiring a perpetual critique of any formulation of a human norm or ideal of "wholeness," is ethical, or, in Mary Daly's language, metaethical. That is, it requires an awareness of issues of justice and oppression, however hard-edged they feel in the soft embrace of the amoral, apolitical insinuation of wholeness. The point, however, is in no way to reduce the spiritual and emotional fullness of the ideal to a moral and political concern, but rather to see beyond the dichotomy of massively social and profoundly individual consummations. Jung's notion of wholeness as conscious attunement with a collective psyche, or unconscious, suggests the ultimate impossibility of the dichotomy, as does--in an altogether different vein, the feminist motto that "the personal is the political."

Rich's imagery, from "Integrity," of the wild patience that makes for completeness; an integrity of "selves":

> Anger and tenderness: the spider's genius
> to spin and weave in the same action
> from her own body, anywhere--
> even from a broken web.

A delicacy of work on self and world is evoked--a willingness to begin from the brokenness, to create rather than wait, like poor Humpty, for the king's men. And it is most important to note, when our topic pertains to "spirit," that the body here--characteristic of feminism--serves as metaphoric vehicle and as a basis of activity, precluding the typical spirit-body dualism that the classical notions of self-realization have bolstered.

Because of the importance of some notion of unbroken selfhood for feminist sensibility, I want to discuss three dangers I discern--for women and therefore for wholeness itself--in the very idea of "wholeness." For certain ways of employing the concept can prove as ineffectual in the process of piecing together as all the king's horses and all the king's men.

(1) Wholeness has come through the Jungian and popular-mythological psychology to imply a complementary union of "masculine" and "feminine," as the primordial opposites, both in relationship and within the individual psyche. There, the true focus of wholeness, it is said to take the form of "androgyny." Many feminists, Daly in _Beyond God the Father_ included, have found the image of the mythic man-woman liberating at a certain stage, suggestive of a plentitude of possibilities beyond traditional gender types and roles. Men could be gentle and nurturant and poetic, as well as strong and directive and analytical--and vice versa. This is all very well, but somewhere along the way the vice versa rebelled, and another verse from Rich turned into a normative declaration:

> These are words I cannot choose again
> _humanism androgyny_
> Such words have no shame in them
> no diffidence before

the raging stoic grandmothers
(from "Natural Resources," same as epigraph).

Androgyny and its wholeness began to smack of an easy theoretical solution that evaded the real issue: the historical loss of a meaningful self-definition for half the race. The way we understand "masculine" and "feminine" is predicated upon this loss and its accompanying compensations. They are stereotypes mascarading (as Nelle Morton has been insistently reminding, asking for a fundamental differentiation) as archetypes. The full dimensionality of egg, womb, web is flattened in stereotype--which means a solid mold used for printing, and so a two-dimensional, static reproduction from a mold which is itself taken from an original mold. It is precisely this static redundancy which, in any form, must be prevented from molding "wholeness."

It may indeed be obfuscation with "no shame" to imagine that we could abstract from a history of stereotypic repetitiveness any sort of essence of both genders, only to add them back together to get wholeness. For male experience in a patriarchy is surely not a matter of one-sided or overstated masculinity. Let me stress this point, for it goes directly against a prevailing way of naming patriarchy as simply a masculine world, or a male dominance in the sense of absence of female participation. I believe this would provide too dismal a picture of male "nature" to allow any hope, and hope is essential to revolution. No, male dominance is not simply unalloyed masculinity, but masculinity gone bad, like a cancerous growth. It is a complex psychosocial pattern completely parasitical upon the subservient and supportive status of women. Female experience within its context has taken the form either of an internalized misogyny refracted in a mirror-game of self-loathing and male-dependency, or an altogether unfeminine, raging stoicism. So we have now a dawning awareness that we must start, if not ex nihilo, from scratch--the scratchy, broken history that women can claim. Otherwise it remains his-story: the feminine from the man's perspective, symbolizing to him his stifled flesh or his lost soul, abhorred or adored, but his.

Androgyny presupposes such masculinity and femininity. In its intention, the overcoming of patriarchy at every level is certainly prefigured, and so its use by Plato, by the Gnostics and alchemists, by psychologists and feminists and writers like Virginia Woolf, should by no means be belittled, flattened. Now it is recognized as too overloaded with assumptions to fulfill its own intention: a powerful symbol ready to die because ready to be realized? The idea of wholeness has not only been elaborated quite often in terms of androgyny, or some such sexual synthesis, but shares in the problematic generality of all such nominous generalities, like "humanism," or "human liberation." Generalization easily serves high-minded avoidance and denial. Yet if wholeness is emptied of the filling of sexual complementarity, the union of opposed stereotypes, it may at suitable moments reveal something of woman's collective desire: for a strength, focus, decisiveness, mobility and will that is not a cancerous "masculine" growth, a psychic penis appended to the female soul; but this is a genuinely womanly strength, a female art of focus and decisiveness, a will arising out of the experience of our selves as women and finally moving free of the inhibitions of self-consciousness and narcissistic mirror-games.

And surely vice versa--that strength in males take the shape of tenderness, that analysis not be merely complemented by creativity, that sensitivity not be viewed as a "feminine" quality, but find, in men, marvelously male gestalts. And furthermore, it is high time that men realized that feminism has no desire for weak men who turn women into mothers; who fear the powers of anger and eros and timidly repress them, rather than engaging in experiments toward a hearing, heedful, expressive and daring rhythm of integrity and passion. Some of this may well be learned through the initiative of women, but cannot depend upon communication with women as women are no longer depending for intimacy and insight upon communication with men. To call such a development an inculcation of "feminine" qualities seems to me increasingly unhelpful. Wholeness, unlike "androgyny," must emerge from the painful integrities of our own gender, our broken web; our alienated bodies.

(2) The second danger I will discuss briefly: it would involve the amplification of certain traditionally feminine attributes into a religious totality, rather than the synthesis of masculine and feminine. This connotation of wholeness is not so much an individual integrity but a loss of self in apparently larger wholes. Wholeness can suggest a psychological state of quiescence, of rest, of passivity, of an achieved equilibrium or harmony, that merely reinforces the most self-defeating traits of a dominated group. It is doubtful that they are traits to be emphasized at the cost of the dynamic, decisive transcendence more associated with masculine possibilities, either for women or men. What Simone de Beauvoir called "immanence" may indeed contain certain values that she herself did not

see, as she focused on the dangers: the temptations therein for abdication of the responsibility of being a self, the temptation to acquiesce in one's otherness and in definition by the imposed circumstances (inevitably patriarchal in our history) remain acute. And in terms of the psychology of women, the fixation on any "wholeness" not carefully assessed, or felt-through, does seem to lead to this inactivity. It can glorify the balancing acts of self-division and relational schism that women have been immersed in all along. Then web-entrapment precludes web-weaving. Wholeness can constitute a genuine temptation to self-loss by its appeal to the classical religious and mystical admonitions to loss of self as a way of finding God, peace, bliss or self itself. Theological feminists like Daly, Ruether, Plaskow speak in unison against the ideal of self-sacrifice, self-loss as viable for the underdeveloped ego-structure of women, whose self-sacrifice as wife and mother has hardly expressed the heights of spiritual freedom. Whether self-sacrifice, self-loss or self-denial in the name of a higher wholeness constitute a healthy ideal for persons in general is another issue to be considered. But in terms of feminism, it is important for us to discern the subtle, wavering line between the passivity of the oppressed, however peaceful the adaption for survival might seem; and the radical creativity that requires a redemption of the receptive, the yin, the relational, the bodily-emotive-intuitive (the litany of the Other Side) from its oppression and repression by the dominant activism. This activism, at best rationalism and at worst simple violence, represents the crude imposition of boundaries upon experience under the reign of the king and his horsemen. It is not the activity of the spider.

This second danger of apparent wholeness, I would want to claim, represents precisely the brokenness from herself and her sister selves of woman after the "great fall." It has been, still is, quite deceptive, for it appeals to our complacency, and yet also to our necessary allegiance to our previous selves.

(3) Under the third danger I wish to subsume this entire thought: for it accounts for the condition of brokenness, the state of male dominance, and the interdependence of the two. Thus it would underlie the polarization of "masculine" and "feminine" that is displayed both in the wholeness of androgyny and of the simple feminine.

Wholeness, I suggested, presupposes brokenness. It means, rather than a guaranteed or essential oneness of some sort, as in a philosophically "simple" unity, an unbroken state: that is, either once broken or at least breakable. Thus there is a realism implicit in the concept which well suits woman's state, in which brokenness is painfully presupposed, whether raging, bleeding or mending. By any therapeutic or theological assessment of culture itself, such presupposed brokenness is true in general. We would not want to jump too rapidly to conclusions about "original sin": but some sort of "great fall" haunts world myth as well as nursery rhymes for a reason.

If there has been a great fall, a great alienation and break, it must be recognized and in that sense presupposed as ever after affecting everything--as the past does. But it can be presupposed also in the sense of a prerequisite: something that is actually required for "wholeness." This latter form of presupposition is quite suspicious, for if perchance the great fall itself was thus required by the King, then the King's men, whether philosophers, therapists or theologians, could never put Humpty together again. They would unconsciously reiterate the brokenness.

Something like this futile cycle threatens the notion of wholeness, for it presupposes a break, a separation, in such a way as to recapitulate the fall as a means to the end, the telos, which is in biblical terms teleios, perfection or completeness. Inasmuch as the self, whether its wholeness is realized or not, is regarded as a separate, independent, self-contained individual, its integrity is based upon an onto-psychological break. And let me further claim that it is no accident that such independence from the inner and outer Other has been the province of male egos. Here is the impatience of my thesis: this fundamental break is won at the expense of woman, for it constitutes a oneness based on an impossible tension of separation from woman as Mother and conquest of woman as Other.

I want to draw upon Jung's concept of wholeness as a paradigm of the dilemma. His articulation of wholeness as the end of psychic growth has shaped all work in the psychology of religion since. Wholeness for him is the aim of the process of individuation, which consists in a series of psychic events regarding the opposites into which the psyche is divided. Consciousness and unconsciousness, masculine and feminine, rationality and spirit suggest the familiar pairs. The divisive character of the ego, as the principle of differentiation, necessitates, or makes possible, the process of dynamic reconciliation. The ego breaks the egg-like unity of unconsciousness. Because the female element represents not only the anima opposite of the male ego but the original womb-like matrix of consciousness, the collective unconscious itself, differentiation and ego-development is fundamentally a process of radical separation from the Mother. Wholeness, then, for Jung is symbolized most adequately by a reconciliation with her--with the entire transpersonal matrix of psychic life beyond the control of the ego. It is quite understandable that has exercised such attraction for women in this century.

I have no desire to dispute the tremendous richness and viability of the Jungian discovery of ranges of psychic experience far deeper than the marshes of id already reclaimed in the Freudian revolution. The notion of wholeness is correspondingly enlarged: for Freud integrity could be centered only in the controlling ego. According to Jung: "For the experience of wholeness, there can be no question of anything cheaper or less than just the whole." This whole is the totality he calls Self: a spirit-center, indeed the Spirit, to which the ego sacrifices itself if individuation is to occur. Yet this sacrifice is meaningless without the prior development of ego.

At this point the psychic futility suggests itself. The ego according to Jung develops, emerges, under the aegis of the symbol of the warrior-Hero--that unabashedly masculine image of the conscious "I." It represents identity as separation and differentiation. For him consciousness is based upon the symbolic matricide mythically imaged in Marduk's "heroic" slaughter of the great mother Tiamat, the oceanic creatrix, through whose conquest Marduk becomes King of the cosmos. "To challenge the unformed chaotic Tiamat world is in fact the primordial experience . . . When man lays his hand to this work, he repeats, as the alchemists say, the creative work of God." Quite so. For Tiamat, whose demise can only euphemistically be described as a "challenge," is the Mesopotamian ancestress of the Hebrew Tehom, "the depths" conquered and contained in the reign of YHWH. Or again, elsewhere, Jung says: "The world begins to exist when the individual discovers it. He discovers it when he sacrifices the 'mother,' when he has freed himself from the mists of his unconscious condition within the mother." Jung refers here to the division of experience into subject and object, into ego and other, enabling the discovery of world as object-sphere: in other worlds, the separation from the symbolic Mother models the entire gamut of dualisms.

In Freudian theory the fundamental conflict, the oedipal crisis, is enacted in relation to the father rather than the mother; and both parents have for him a much more literal and personally past reference than they do in Jung's archetypal theory. Yet at this point both can shed light on the structures of misogyny, though Jung, by acknowledging the priority of matricide, hovers much closer, it seems to me, to an understanding of patriarchy. (This does not imply that he seeks its overthrow . . .) According to the symbolism of the heroic matricide, woman as the primordial non-ego would ever after evoke a certain myth-powered ambivalence, a dual forcefield of attraction to the source and the promise of reconciliation, and matriophobic hostility. Woman's psyche receives little direct illumination by Jung's inversions of this scheme. While lending an extremely telling analysis of the cultural psyche, Jung continues to presuppose its fundamental structure as necessity: the separation is necessary for the reconciliation with Her, ad nauseam.

The Freudian model lends insight into the formation of the dualistic object-relations which characterize precisely such an heroically autonomous, separate psyche. For while the fundamental conflict is depicted as patricidal, it in fact represents a "smashing of the pre-oedipal bond to the mother." In "Mermaid and the Minotaur," Dorothy Dinnerstein, a feminist neo-Freudian, has shown how this original break is then ever recapitulated in the relations of men and women to women--inasmuch as an independent ego is to be achieved. She does not challenge this deeper point, the point which I consider the third danger of wholeness: the necessity for a primal break as means of differentiating self and other into the separate entities of a dualistic world-view. She suggests equal early childcare by male and female in order to distribute the residual hostility of separation equally between the sexes, thus relieving the psychic need for misogyny. But is it not possible that the need for separation--rather than stretching, distancing and differentiating within a continuum--is what finally needs to be questioned?

Nancy Chodorow, another neo-Freudian, suggests a new look at the nature of the pre-oedipal bond, whether or not it could be equally attached to the father. She suggests that precisely because the female child is not required in our (heroic) culture to accomplish a complete separateness of identity, she experiences herself as "continuous with others" (Reproduction of Mothering). Growing girls' "experience of self contains more flexible or permeable ego boundaries. Boys come to define themselves as more separate and distinct, with a greater sense of rigid ego boundaries and differentiation. The basic feminine sense of self is connected to the world, the basic masculine sense of self is separate" (169). The sense of self refers for her both to inner and outer object relations.

Conclusion

Pieced together, these are important clues, I hope, as to possible pitfalls in the notion of wholeness. For wholeness, while it may represent a reconciliation with the "mother," the "feminine," it suggests a vertical depth which in no fundamental sense includes the world. If wholeness, to be that, cannot stop at "anything cheaper or less than just the whole," it must as a concept include an essential reference to the presence of all things in all things: not as an afterthought, as when we add together "inner and outer," or "inter- and intra-personal" to make clear we mean all the proper social contexts, however. It must find its way into the very thinking about what it is to be unbroken. Otherwise wholeness remains predicated upon the structure of the separate-masculine-ego, and its attempts to recover the world will resemble conquest or inflation. (Thus Jung's work remains vulnerable to accusations of individualism.) Individuality refers semantically to an undividedness: and perhaps we can begin to think this undividedness as much more than an internal unification that basically excludes the Other, but as a state of being undivided from the universe. To be unbroken from the totality--yet not therefore merged into a spuriously simple unity of self-loss with it. The break from the matrix is the fundamental antic of the hero, a swordsman's gesture to be repeated with ontic consequence. Once separated from the inflowing presences of the world at large, the source of replenishment for soul is cut off. Then, sameness of identity, a redundant attempt to approximate permanence and a controlling, unifying center increase in importance. Even spirit, with its original play of breath, of windy lightness and gusty power, becomes against all likelihood something fixed, an unmoving center, a King.

The simple unity of the egg cannot be regained, culturally or individually, ever--it is the ever inchoate source of things, the matrix too enormous for consciousness. Consciousness is always within, arising from, this encompassing surroundment. The attempt to regain this primal unity seems to lie behind the ideal of androgyny and the glorification of the feminine as compensation for some cosmic loss--loss, indeed, of cosmos. Such a regressive attempt requires the image of the waiting woman, embracing the returning hero: he who has separated subject from object, conscious from unconscious, ego from self, with his frantic swordsmanship, and now seeks frantically, with the same crude tool, to put the original connection back together again. Wholeness, unless it is to lack the subtle activism of the spider's spinning from the given toward the new, unless it is to forfeit all ethical and therefore value-transformative and consciousness-shaping claims, must divest itself of psychic nostalgia of this sort. Otherwise woman's self remains submerged in the other, man's self subsumes the other, and we learn nothing of the arising from other, the issue into other, which sets the cadence of the self's moment-by-moment emergence and perishing. We cannot learn about the concatenation and internal communing of selves, suggested not only by the poet Rich, but by Buddhism, by Whitehead, by Santayana and Gurdjieff, among others, which would break up the illusion of a static wholeness of identity itself won through a perpetual breakage.

The "wild patience" of the arachnid opus of integrity obviates the futile gestures of the king's men. A new whole always, never an old egg! Still, the image of the cosmic egg emerges at a vital point in women's literature, a point of intersection of the personal and the political in the apocalyptic symbolism of Doris Lessing's Memoirs of a Survivor. At the end of this work and of the world it depicts, a small community of selves, strangely part of each other's present and of each other's memories, both sexes and three generations, are together "in that place which might present us with anything . . . " They are in the presence of a giant black egg. "There they stood, looking at this iron egg until, broken by the force of their being there, it fell apart, and out it came . . . "

Far be it from me to give away the plot of the end of the world. If as Jung suggested the world is created by a matricide, then that world's end must be the end, the telos, of wholeness. Wild patience is tender, angry and psychosocially apocalyptic.

References

Athanassak, Apoostolos N., trans. The Homeric Hymns. Baltimore: Johns Hopkins University Press, 1976.

Bachofen, J. J. Myth, Religion & Mother Right: Selected Writings. Princeton: University Press, Bollingen Series 84, paperback edition, 1973.

Brindel, June Rachuy. Ariadne: A Novel of Ancient Crete. New York: St. Martin's Press, 1980.

Chodorow, N. Reproduction of Mothering: Psychoanalysis and the Sociology of Gender. Berkeley: University of California Press, 1978.

Gimbutas, Marija. Goddesses and Gods of Old Europe 7000-3500 B.C.: Myths, Legends, and Cult Images. Los Angeles: University of California Press, revised 1980.

Griffin, Susan. Woman and Nature: The Roaring Inside Her. New York: Harper and Row, 1978.

Harrison, Jane Ellen. Prolegomena to the Study of Greek Religion. 1903; reprint. New York: Meridian Books, 1955.

Jung, C. G. Psychology and Religion: West and East. New York: Bollingen Foundation, 1958.

Kereni, K. Eleusis, Archetypal Image of Mother and Daughter. Trans. Ralph Manheim. 1967; reprint. New York: Schocken Books, 1977.

RELATIONAL WHOLENESS

Whole Holiness--Holy Wholeness: The Interface of Spiritual and Mental Health

H. Newton Malony

Bear Bryant and Nicholas Hobbs are dead. Within a month after he resigned as football coach of Alabama, Bear Bryant died. Within three weeks of attending the ceremony naming a building in his honor, Nicholas Hobbs died. Both men exemplified an essential aspect of wholeness and holiness--they cared for others.

Many of his players remembered Bear Bryant as a coach who built character as well as football teams. They felt loved by him. They mourned his death as one who played a father role in their lives. Nicholas Hobbs, in turn, never forgot a name. He would ask about your spouse by name even if he had not seen you for years. His students used to say, "We believe in the Father, the Son, the Holy Ghost AND in Nicholas Hobbs." Yes, Bryant and Hobbs were holy and whole in the sense that they cared about other people.

Yet neither man was conventionally religious. Although Hobbs was a Unitarian and although Bryant's funeral took place in a Methodist church, conventional religion was not their forte. How, then, can it be said that they were "holy"? The answer is simple. Being holy is not the same as being religious in the customary sense. Much conventional religion is not holy as thinkers from Amos to Kierkegaard have noted. The prophet Micah stated it well by suggesting that the divine imperative requires that one "do justly, love mercy, and to walk humbly with . . . God" (6:8). All other religion implies "cheap grace," as Kierkegaard was wont to say. Neither Bryant nor Hobbs could be accused of cheap religion. Their concern for others was deep and long-standing. Mourners were encouraged to give money for the treatment of disturbed children--a passion of psychologist Hobbs alongside his proclivity for remembering people's names. Those who worked with and played for Bryant were attracted to him because of his reputation of concern for persons off, as well as on, the football field.

At times, mental health has been thought to be an inner quality which existed apart from an outer concern for the welfare of others. Similarly, spiritual health has sometimes been pictured as a private state of inner peace divorced from deeds of loving kindness. Neither of these is true. Becoming whole in terms of mental health or holy in terms of spiritual health is only achieved when persons turn their attention away from self-preoccupation and become invested in the lives of other persons. Both wholeness and holiness have a social and ethical meaning which cannot be ignored.

Without doubt, certain kinds of health can exist apart from service to others, but OPTIMAL mental or spiritual health cannot. To illustrate, there are, at least, three understandings of health: the negative, the normal, and the positive. Negative health means the absence of disease. An example would be the person who says, "I'm well. I got rid of my stomach virus." Normal health means the ability to function about as well as anybody else. An example would be the person who says, "I weigh within a few pounds of the average person my age, and I don't get any more fatigued than the next guy." Positive health means the achievement of some ideal goal. An example would be the person who states, "I finally ran the 10 kilometer race, and I feel better than I ever felt in my life!" This last is the OPTIMAL understanding of health. It is to this definition that my statement about service to others would apply. One cannot be optimally healthy in either a spiritual or a mental manner unless and until one becomes unselfishly concerned with the welfare of others. This is what it means to be whole and to be holy. Of course, there are other components of ideal health, but selfless service is an essential ingredient.

I do not believe that the process of healing is complete until a person has found a channel for using his/her energies in helping others. Getting well or feeling good can never be ends in themselves. In the final analysis, they must serve higher purposes. As Plato suggested, both health and happiness are "secondary" virtues. They can never be primary. It is what one DOES with health that is most important. And humanitarian concern is among the highest of virtues.

Elsewhere I have written about this optimal understanding of healing under the rubric of the ALABAMA model of psychotherapy (Collins and Malony, 1981). Herein, the "As" (affirmations of faith) guide my response to the "L" (the life situation), and the "Bs" (the background variables) as well as to my use of the "M" (my therapeutic model). One of these "As" is the presumption that the task of psychotherapy is not complete until a person comes to know him/herself as a child of God (deeply loved and completely forgiven) AND has found a ministry of service to others. Obviously, this is an ideal definition of the psychotherapeutic process that goes beyond the alleviation of symptoms and beyond average adjustment to the environment. An achievement of an optimal state is implied. Although the typical psychotherapeutic relationship is problem-centered and usually ends when those problems of living are solved, this does not detract in the least from the ideal state of affairs in which persons go beyond their preoccupation with problems and become concerned with the purpose of life. And I am convinced that the TRUE purpose of life includes an investment in other human beings.

In addition to being content with problem-solving, psychotherapy can become distorted by an overconcern with feelings of well-being. This can be seen in much of the holistic health writings where spiritual and mental health are often understood as complete when one has achieved a deep sense of inner harmony coupled with excellent physical health resulting from exercise and diet. Much energy is put into meditation, imaging, healthful food, and self-control. The more one accomplishes this harmony of body, mind and spirit, the healthier one is.

However this is a <u>state</u>, instead of a <u>trait</u> theory of health, and states of mind can never substitute for traits of behavior. I believe, like William James, that health should be judged by its fruits--what it produces in actual behavior. An example of this distortion was a recent address given by a holistic health physician. He displayed elaborate diagrams depicting the proper balance of thought, feeling and physique. He even included a section on harmonious interpersonal relationships. Toward the end of his address he showed slides of his newly established retreat in the forest of a South American country to which he invited all seekers of holistic health. Although he may have intended to say something about it, I strongly doubt whether his understanding of health included any responsibility for the natives who struggled for existence in that environment that he considered so idyllic or whether his understanding included any returns to the mainland from which he was fleeing except to recruit more persons to join him in his Shangri-la.

Participants in such retreat centers may have the STATE of health, but I question whether they exhibit the TRAIT of health. Health, as noted earlier, is simply a preparation for action. It cannot be an end in itself. As Jesus reminded us, we are to love others as we love ourselves (Luke 10:27). And in many situations about the only neighbor that is "loved" is the person sitting next to one in a circle uttering his/her "OM" in identical narcissistic preoccupation. Such is not health from an ideal point of view.

Paul Vitz would term this type of self-centeredness "psychology AS religion" (1977) in the sense that persons mistakenly perceive their own sense of well-being to be the highest value in their lives. From an ideal point of view, this is highly questionable. I do not believe this to be good psychology, much less good religion. At best, many of the understandings of holistic health appear to me to be NORMAL, but not IDEAL, definitions of health. Since they seem to omit a strong concern for others' welfare, I do not consider them to be whole or holy. They do not reflect optimal states of either mental or spiritual health.

As the famous Harvard psychologist Henry Murray suggested in comparing outward and inward spirals of life, those who move inward toward themselves are moving toward mental illness, while those who move outward toward others are moving toward mental health. William Booth, the founder of the Salvation Army, reportedly decided to send a Christmas greeting to all of the Salvation Army workers throughout the world. When he found that his original greeting was too expensive, he asked what would be the cost of a ten-word greeting. This, too, was too expensive. Finally he settled on a one-word telegram that would not cost too much yet would convey the essence of their mission. It was "Others." Kirk Farnsworth, in writing about the relationship between psychology and theology, termed a concern for others "embodied integration" (1982), as if to say, "the best combination of mental and spiritual health can be found in persons who embody (or evidence) inner harmony and outer concern for others."

In this regard, it is of interest to note that in a recent article in Psychology Today on "What makes a top executive?", the primary characteristic of those who failed was "an abrasive, bullying style which reflected an insensitivity to other people" (McCall and Lombardo, 1983, p. 28). In contrast to this, a successful young Australian business executive said recently, "When I retire I will have considered myself successful if those who worked under me report that I helped them fulfill their potentials and life goals." Although he, like any other chief executive officer, reads with keen interest the loss/profit column at the end of each fiscal year, it is noteworthy that he judged his effectiveness on the basis of his impact on persons--not on products.

Earlier in this essay, it was suggested that Bear Bryant and Nicholas Hobbs embodied, or evidenced, this quality of concern for others, but that it was divorced from conventional religion. So was the aforementioned business executive's attitude toward his employees. However, it was also suggested earlier that TRUE religion included this dimension whether it was conventional or not. The lack of a necessary connection between explicit religious ideology and true spirituality was affirmed by Oden (1965) in his discussion of the use of theological terms in psychotherapy. His point of view has been termed "implicit Christology." He concluded that when the therapist provided optimal conditions of empathy, congruence and warmth, the conditions of Christ's incarnation were present and that God was active and present in the situation. Neither God's name nor the religious meaning of the moment had to be said. God was present whether his presence was made verbally explicit or not.

So with unselfish behavior. God's will is being done whether this is stated or not. If by spiritual health we mean doing the will of God, then those who care for others are evidencing a degree of spiritual health whether they know it or not.

If it be true, as Wilson (1975) and other sociobiologists have concluded, that altruism is embedded in the genes, then service to others is not a radical ethical decision made in the face of egotism, but, rather, the outworking of a tendency inherent in human nature itself. The typical theological assertion that only human decision can bridge the gap between the "is" and the"ought" (cf. Nelson, 1980) may be incorrect. The possibility that social ethics is a genetic tendency would make mental and spiritual health (wholeness and holiness) one, not two, ideals--as many have assumed them to be. Of course, such a conclusion would entail according legitimacy to the contention that (1) there is a spiritual reality in which humans live which is as objectively real as their physical environment, and (2) that humans are innately capable of responding to that reality by virtue of the way in which they were created.

There is some warrant for concluding that the organ through which these physical/spiritual realities are mediated is the brain. The brain may be a repository of human capacities to interact with both empirical and transempirical environments. Soul may simply be a term for the cranial ability to respond to the transcendent. MIND may be an encompassing term for the expression of this combined interaction. And the health of the mind may be a function of the extent to which it reflects a response to the spiritual as well as the physical world.

Certainly this was the contention of Augustine and Jung. Augustine's famous statement, "Thou hast made us for thyself and our hearts are restless until they find their rest in thee" is a succinct statement of this point of view. Paul, writing in Romans, espoused this idea when he stated, "When Gentiles, who have not the law do by nature what the law requires, they are a law unto themselves, even though they do not have the law. They show that what the law requires is written on their hearts . . . " (2:14-15a, RSV).

And Carl Jung's dictum that neurosis in persons over thirty-five was most often due to persons being cut off from the spiritual world of which the world's great religions spoke is further testimony to this idea. "No man, Jung maintained, can lead a truly adequate life relating only to the material world; we also need to be in contact with the divine reality that is superior to us. One is stupid, dull, or neurotic if not in touch with that reality. In other words, religion is not some perfume we add to an already adequate and well scrubbed life. It is necessary to an adequate life" (Kelsey, 1982, p. 16). Humans are, indeed, "amphibious creatures" who can, and should, relate to both the physical AND the spiritual realms of reality, according to Kelsey. Sarbin's (1970) proposal that humans have to relate to the self-maintenance, the social, the normative AS WELL AS the transcendent ecologies if they would be fully functioning is further proof of this interrelationship between mental and spiritual health.

In another essay entitled "Wholeness and Holiness" (1983), I suggested that persons' response to the transcendent ecology transformed in a multiplicative manner their interactions with the other environments of their lives. This attaches a prime importance to transcendent reality in the sense that here it is possible for persons to find the security that makes it possible for them to sustain the interest in others which characterized such lives as those of Bear Bryant and Nicholas Hobbs. In reactions to all of the other ecologies, persons are primarily motivated by their own survival and self-interest.

This effect has been succinctly described by Duncombe in The Shape of the Christian Life. He suggests that the overarching effect of becoming a Christian (or establishing a relationship with the transcendent ecology) is that it gives a person "a freeing sense of security." Subsequently there are four other effects according to Duncombe: self-knowledge, accurate perception, honest expression, and adequate response. These are diagrammed by Duncombe in the following manner which co-varies active and passive modes and subjective and objective perspectives (p. 22).

RESULTS OF THE CHRISTIAN LIFE
A FREEING SENSE OF SECURITY AND ITS
FOUR IDENTIFYING CHARACTERISTICS

A Freeing Sense of Security

To live with the kind of inner freedom, both normally and in the face of threat or uncertainty, that has no need to distort or manipulate life to make it seem more secure

	Self Knowledge	Accurate Perception
Passive Modality (perceiving)	The ability to recognize and acknowledge as one's own those past and present thoughts, feelings, and acts which most deeply affect one's life.	The ability to perceive the world as it is, to have a sensitive awareness of others' lives, and to be open to all kinds of experiences.
	Honest Expression	Adequate Response
Active Modality (responding)	The ability to express one's desires, feelings, thoughts, and doubts naturally and without fear.	The ability to respond in a way appropriate to the nature and occasion of that which is experienced, adopting behavioral patterns not bound by personal scruples or social expectations.
	Subjective Perspective	Objective Perspective

These are <u>psychological</u> results of a <u>theological</u> process in the sense that the results of becoming a Christian are described in terms of inner perceptions and outer behaviors rather than in terms of eternal salvation or status with God. This reinforces my contention that wholeness and holiness are intricately interrelated. Holiness was implicitly present in the wholeness seen in Bryant and Hobbs. So in Duncombe's model. Wholeness is present in the holiness that comes from true Christianity.

Duncombe's model warrants a closer examination. The central theme is FREEDOM; the prime effect of becoming a Christian is to have a "freeing sense of security." Paul spoke of this experience of freedom through a comparison of Abraham's two sons--one of whom was born to a slave and the other to Sarah, his wife. Using this story allegorically, he suggested that those who followed the Jewish law were "children of bondage," while those who followed him were free. In a dramatic plea, he stated, "Freedom is what we have--Christ has set us free! Stand, then, as free men, and do not allow yourselves to become slaves again" (Galatians 5:1, TEV).

Psychologically this freedom is freedom from the desperate, frantic attempt to prove one's self-worth to God or to other people. As Duncombe suggested, it is a "freeing sense of security" that allows one to live without distortion or manipulation--both of which would be efforts to assure the security that best comes from faith. Bondage to the law, as Paul conceived it, was just that. It was a conviction that God was an unforgiving judge who weighed the worth of persons on a scale of obedience and good works. It was the conviction that one was never fully secure and that one had to keep diligently proving oneself. This was the essence of sin, according to Paul. It was tantamount to belief in the wrong kind of God; a belief which, in turn, led to a desperate type of existence.

This interface between faith and life, which I have termed the interrelation between wholeness and holiness or mental and spiritual health, is clearly portrayed in Duncombe's model of the four settings of existence. These settings are easily recognizable as the arenas in which one interacts with inner experience and outer reality. In turn, these settings have both an awareness and an expressive dimension to them in the sense that, as human beings, we are always able to think about, as well as respond to, events.

The first of Duncombe's four depictions of the results of Christian faith suggests that in the arena of self-awareness, the Christian is able to admit into consciousness all those thoughts, feelings, and actions which have made the person who he/she is coupled with the ability to honor this life-experience without denial or omission. This is to say, for the Christian there is enough inner security to say to oneself, "I am who I am. It's OK to be me."

The second of Duncombe's descriptions of the effects of Christian faith refers to the environmental arena. The Christian can perceive the world as it is and is free enough from his/her own inner demands for recognition and status so that new experiences are not threatening, and other's needs are not ignored. In the terms of Transactional Analysis, this means, "I'm OK and You're OK." There is only one qualification: the Christian also recognizes evil when s/he sees it and does not pretend that there are no problems when there are.

The third result of being Christian which Duncombe mentions occurs in the arena of self-expression. Here faith results in openness and honesty with others. The Christian does not hold back or calculate. Because the deep needs for recognition and status have been settled once and for all through faith, there is no continuing need to suppress one's feelings or deny one's thoughts. There is the confidence that one will be accepted because one has been accepted.

The fourth, and final, result of Christian faith has to do with persons' behaviors in the world. Duncombe's term for this is "adequate response." Here the Christian does what should be done. Action is neither held back nor impulsive but, in a mysterious way, is appropriate to the occasion and has an impact on others apart from custom or opinions. Once again, the Christian is not primarily motivated by his/her own need for social security or acceptance, but, because of faith, has the freedom to do what is good in an ultimate sense. It is here that the Christian joins in acts for peace and justice with the confidence that this is the will of God for human beings.

In response to the above descriptions some people might say, "This is utterly idealistic. It has no meaning for everyday life." The first statement is true; the second is false. These are, indeed, IDEAL descriptions of what SHOULD be the results of faith if faith was fully effective. As was noted earlier, that is the nature of holiness or wholeness when it is conceived positively rather than normally or negatively. It is perfectly legitimate to propose ideal definitions for these states even though they are rarely achieved and even though they must always be contextualized in specific situations.

This leads me to the second statement that such ideal understandings of wholeness and holiness have no relevance to daily life. I disagree. Ideals always hover over us, and while they may never be fully actualized, they do influence who we are and what we do. The possibility that faith will provide a sense of freedom, full self-knowledge, accurate perception, honest expression, and adequate response functions like a lighthouse for sailors at sea. Although their route may deviate in an idiosyncratic manner along the channel, they yet look to the lighthouse for guidance and reassurance both in calm and stormy conditions. It may be difficult to show how the lighthouse determined the route of a particular ship, but its influence would be there just the same.

An example of this impact can be seen in a recent study entitled "Health and Holiness: An Examination of the Relationship between Self-Concept and the Perception of Christ's Ethics" (Raney and Malony, 1983). A group of college students, all of whom identified themselves as Christians, were classified by testing as having low or high self-esteem. They were subjected to an experiment in which they were required to make one of two choices in a total of 40 situations. They were rewarded by chips which they could exchange for changes in a $100 lottery. The situations afforded them the chance to be increasingly self-denying. Halfway through the experiment, they were told to make the rest of their choices on the basis of what they thought Christ would do in that situation. Although both groups were more self-denying in the Jesus role than in the self role, those with high self-esteem were less self-denying during the time when they were being themselves and more self-denying during the time when they were trying to behave as Jesus would. These results clearly indicate how the ideal functions in real life and how the effect of being Christian is greater in some persons than others.

Self-esteem is a complex issue, and this study indicates that becoming a Christian does not automatically raise everyone's self-esteem to an identical level. Each person is unique and, while people's self-esteem is no doubt influenced by their faith, each individual has a unique enough history to conclude that the interaction of spiritual and mental health will be an individual one. Nevertheless, it can be said with certainty that ideal understandings of wholeness as well as holiness do have a practical impact on life whether this impact is clearly recognized or not.

This essay has dealt with the interface between mental and spiritual health. It has contended that when health is conceived from a positive, rather than a negative or normal, point of view, there are distinct similarities between the two. In fact, it could be said that while at the negative and normal levels there may be a warrant for separating them, at the positive, or ideal level, mental and spiritual health begin to converge. Wholeness, the term for mental health, may be similar to holiness, the term for spiritual health. Through the examples of Bear Bryant and Nicholas Hobbs and the recounting of David Duncombe's model for the effects of Christian faith, it was demonstrated that the two have common, if not identical, themes. There may be, indeed, such things as "whole holiness" and "holy wholeness"!

References

Collins, G. R., and Malony, H. N. Psychology and Theology: Prospects for Integration. New York: Abingdon Press, 1981.

Duncombe, D. C. The Shape of the Christian Life. New York: Abingdon Press, 1969.

Farnsworth, K. E. "The Conduct of Integration." Journal of Psychology and Theology , 1982, 10(4), 308-319.

Jahoda, M. Current Concepts of Positive Mental Health. New York: Basic Books, 1958.

Kelsey, M. T. Christo-Psychology. New York: Crossroad, 1982.

Malony, H. N. (Ed.). Wholeness and Holiness: Readings in the Psychology/Theology of Mental Health. Grand Rapids, Michigan: Baker Book House, 1983.

McCall, Jr., M. W., and Lombardo, M. M. "What Makes Top Executives?" Psychology Today, 1983 (February), 28-31.

Nelson, J. R. "A Theologian's Response to Wilson's On Human Nature. Zygon, 1980, 15(4), 397-406.

Oden, T. C. Atonement and Psychotherapy. Philadelphia: Westminster Press, 1965.

Raney, R. W., and Malony, H. N. "Health and Holiness: An Examination of the Relationship between Self-Concept and the Perception of Christ's Ethics." Paper presented at the annual meeting of the Christian Association for Psychological Studies, Western Region, San Jose, California, May, 1983.

Sarbin, T. R. "A Role Theory Perspective for Community Psychology: The Structure of Social Identity." In D. Adelson and B. L. Kalis (Eds.) Community Psychology and Mental Health: Perspectives and Challenges. Scranton, Pennsylvania: Chandler Publishing Company, 1970, 89-113.

Vitz, P. C. Psychology as Religion: The Cult of Self Worship. Grand Rapids, Michigan: William B. Eerdman's Company, 1977.

Wilson, E. O. *On Human Nature*. Cambridge, Massachusetts: Harvard University Press, 1978.

Dancing with Notitia: The Spirit Centered Female Core of Knowledge

Moreen Kamiki Cutter Bratt

HOW IMAGES PUSH US TO NOTICING

> Whoever on this earth has seen these is blessed, but they who have no part in the holy rites have another lot as they waste away in dank darkness.
>
> --The Hymn to Demeter--

> Hye! Kye!
>
> --The Eleusinian Mystery--

For me, two symbols bracket the world in which we live: the mushroom cloud arising from a nuclear explosion and the image of earth photographed from space.

The shock of Hiroshima, the shock of the potential of nuclear war not only to end all human lives, but to end the very capacity of earth to sustain life, explodes human imagination, sending imagination into space, sending men to the moon and machines beyond the moon. The men on the moon have found it, as expected, barren of life and battered by cosmic debris. As far as we can reach we find a vast, destructive, hostile, desolate universe.

I turn toward earth. The picture seen knocks the breath out of me. I see a blue and green orb enfolded in clouds. I recognize a tiny planet webbed together by a fragile system, an infinitely complex system which nurtures the miracle of life. Coming down to earth, I imagine standing naked in a wood, drenched by torrents of rain. I imagine touching a red crocus, first flower of spring. I imagine hugging the sweet grass, kissing the muddy dirt, smearing red oil over my body, so glad to be alive, on earth, with plants, with animals, with humans.

If we humans were magically removed from our planet, earth would yet be life-filled. Cycles of life, including arousal, rest, birth, death, decay, and rebirth, would continue. Periodically flowers would bloom, bees work, fruits ripen, birds sing, salmon spawn, hawks play, seas rage, rainbows leap, and storms pass. I call all this the "existential natural world." We humans are born into the scene of the enspirited natural world and often seem to begin life commenting on her. The singing, crying, wide-eyed wonder of the newborn infant is met by the laughing, crying, wide-eyed wonder of the new parents and the entire human community.

However, we humans are also born into the scene of culture, a scene which Kenneth Burke points out is more or less made-up and enacted, and as Claude Levi-Strauss has suggested is also a scene in which existential raw nature has been more or less cooked-up. These components which are human-linked I call the "cultural world of Earth."

Each human being is born into, and more or less experiences, both the existential natural world and the cultural world and more or less mediates the resulting interplay of difference between raw nature and cooked-up culture. We live in a time when culture is over-cooked, too removed from raw nature.

The structural anthropologist Claude Levi-Strauss and the ovular feminist writer Susan Griffin note that in such constructions woman is equated with nature, and man equated with culture. While Levi-Strauss asserts that the equation reflects nature, Griffin, in _Woman and Nature: The Roaring Inside Her_, cites examples from Plato to the present, demonstrating that this notion is cooked up by men. It is the construction of opposites in which half the equation equates woman with nature, darkness, death, finitude, mud, soil, and evil.

Griffin's feminist critique calls us to notice that the cyclical, inclusive character of the existential natural world is subordinated to story. This mud: woman: evil spell diverts effective, substantial cultural change, distorts noticing, drains spirit out of noticing, and dispirits human culture and human individuals. Within the scene of the fiction of opposites and opposition the draining of spirit is more or less overlooked because life and the existential natural world is so enspirited that the existential experience of spirit is constantly replenished. However, from its onset the industrial world has so assaulted and wounded the web of life on Earth that spirit is actually being depleted.

The scene of the specter of nuclear annihilation now calls us to attend to life on Earth. Now, the whole of life on Earth is noticed to be more or less connected and more or less vulnerable. Now, Earth is perceived to be awesomely beautiful and has literally been so seen by all of us.

Thus, we begin to remember our heritage. Now we remember our mother the Earth. As we speak, we see in early pre-literature imagery the personification of Earth in female figures. Our noticing is informed by reading backward from Greek texts which recall some of her myriad names: Gaia, Earth, our mother, she who brings forth, the one whose aspects are many: Demeter, two-fold aspect of the whole, divine mother and divine measure, all gifts and the source of all gifts; Aphrodite, incarnate beauty arising from the foaming sea, signifying the aroused and the arousing; Artemis, she who is one in herself, who gentles wild nature, and who acts as midwife to all living; and Persephone, the underworld aspect of Demeter, mediatrix of death and personification of rebirth.

Though the meaning of these "goddesses" may be unfamiliar, they can be remembered by all of us through careful attention to the word, that is, through the commonsense reading of words. This lock on words is related to the denigration of images, to an abhorrence of reading pictorial images, pretending that words are not delightfully, as well as importantly, ambiguous.

Western education teaches people to read texts but rarely teaches people to read images as texts. Because I have been asked to examine both feminist and cross-cultural perspectives in relation to spirit-centered wholeness, turn with me here to notice another culture, the florescence of ancient Crete, c. 2200-1450 B.C. It is a culture without translated word texts but rich in pictorial material. It is pre-Greek, pre-patriarchal, and pre-Western. Noticing this culture is intended to call the basic recipe of Western culture more or less into question.

NOTICING THE IMAGES[1]

I have chosen characteristic images of ancient Crete made during a long florescence (2200-1450 B.C.):

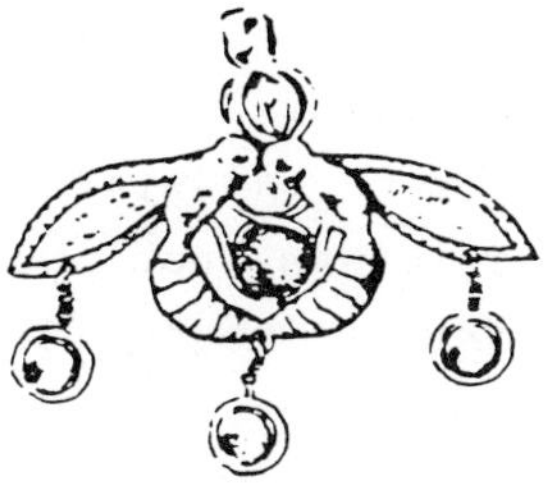

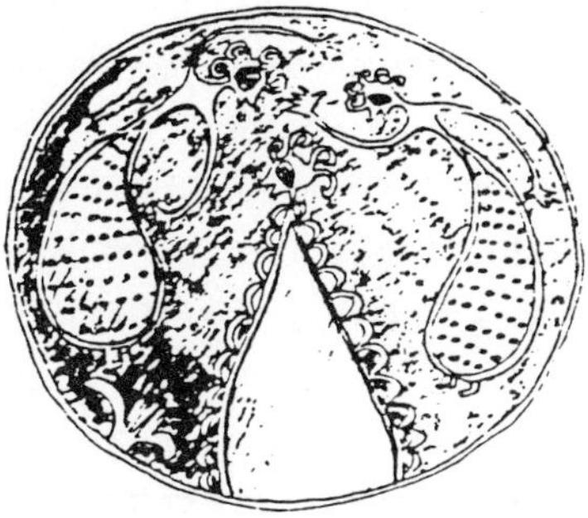

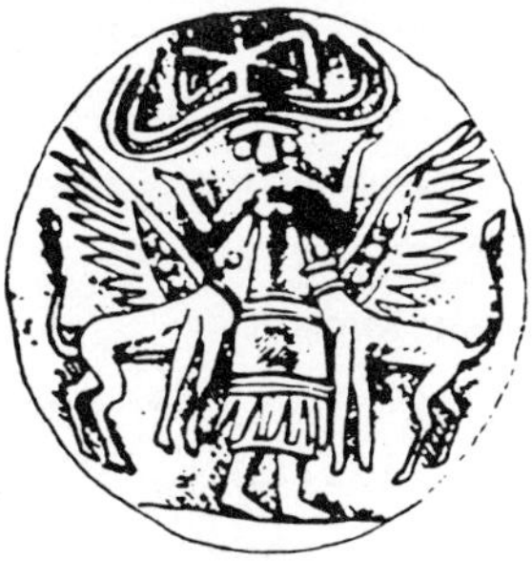

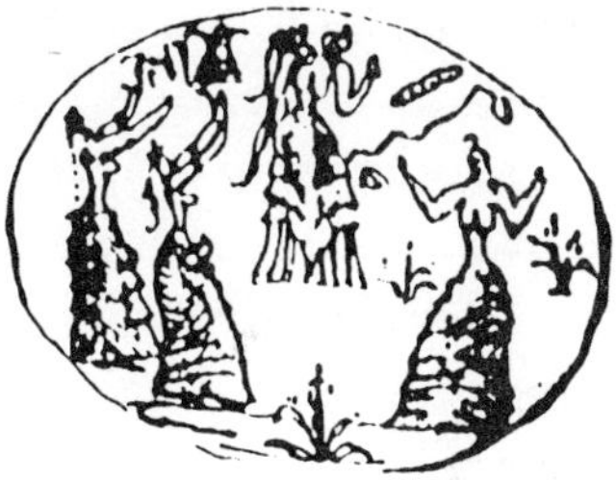

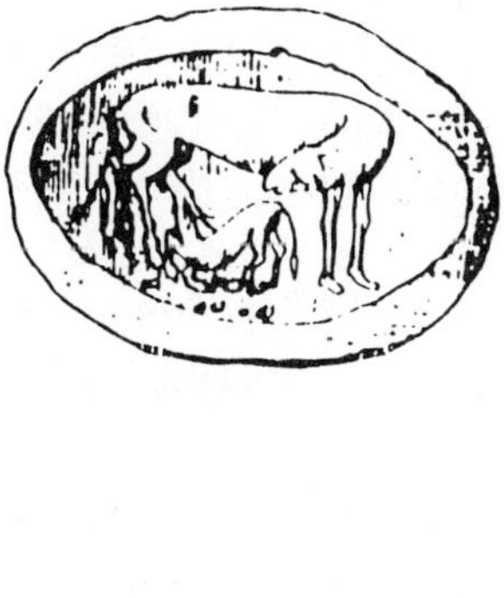

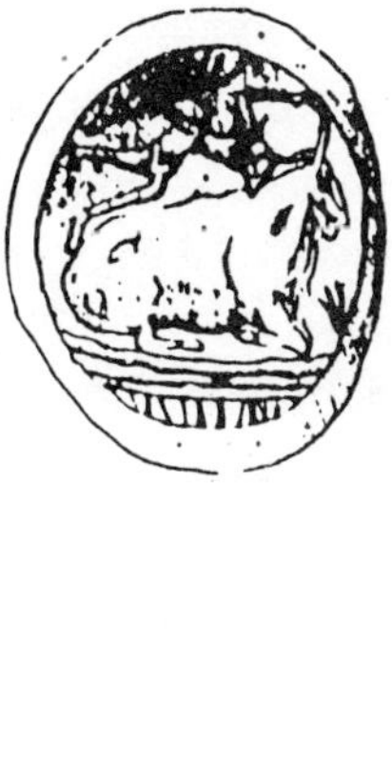

A bull and bull-leaper paired with a cow nursing her calf; a golden pair of bees; a female character emerging from earth flanked by dancing, bee-like characters; bee-headed female characters dancing among flowers; and a central, bee-headed female character flanked by fabulous animals called griffins.

Although the ancient people of Crete had writing, surviving materials are scarce, and it has not been deciphered. However, these ahistorical images from Crete can be read as text. The images can be looked at and described accurately. The images occur in an archeological context which contributes to developing a text from the images.

ATTENTION TO THE CONTEXT OF HISTORY

According to archeologist James Mellaart, people arrived on Crete about 7000 B.C. They brought with them domestic plants and animals, including wheat, barley, sheep, and goats. The people arrived by boat and settled at the site known today as Knossos.

There was continuous occupation of the site with no break in culture until the nearby island of Thera exploded in a violent volcanic eruption around 1450 B.C. After that event, which leveled many architectural structures on Crete, there was a fifty-year occupation of Knossos by Mycenaeans, and then about 1400 B.C. the site was abandoned. Mycenaean overlords stayed on until the twelfth century B.C. when there was a collapse not only of Mycenaean-Greek culture but a general collapse of culture throughout the ancient world.

Throughout the 5500-year cultural continuum on Crete, the imagery is consistently female-centered pointing to a female-centered conceptualization of spirit. In turn, such female-centered concepts seem to enspirit the entire culture, particularly the last five to seven hundred years which are referred to as the flowering of this culture.

The period of cultural climax is usually called Minoan culture, a reference to a Greek myth about a King Minos, which in turn is possibly a reference to a period of Mycenaean-Greek domination or to even later Greek overlords. However, the pre-Greek culture was referred to in contemporaneous texts as the culture of the Keph people. Therefore, I choose to refer to the pre-Greek period as that of Keph culture.

During the period of cultural flowering which began by 2200 B.C., Keph contact was established far and wide with archeological evidence of Keph presence and influence in Egypt, the Levant, and in the heartland of Mycenaean Greek society. Hunt and battle scenes were commonplace in contemporaneous cultures of antiquity. Therefore it is important to observe that although on Crete Keph artisans never illustrated scenes of conflict or war, they did satisfy Mycenaean taste for both hunt and battle scenes.

The Keph people preferred scenes of dancing and organized their great community centers around a central dancing court. The community centers, built during the period of florescence, have been called palaces, but they functioned as working places for artisans, as storage centers, and as ceremonial centers. All were located in places of scenic beauty.

Knossos was the most important. At Knossos the "dancing court" was located directly over the original Neolithic village site. In contrast with Mycenaean architecture which imposed one plan on every terrain,

Keph structures evolved organically, more or less in a structural spiral around a sacred core, replicating the concept of sacred center.

Keph culture collapsed suddenly following the catastrophic volcanic destruction of the nearby island of Thera. Just at the time of the explosion weapons appeared on Crete for the first time. It seems reasonable that the armed Mycenaean soldiers, illustrated in wall paintings at a Keph settlement on Thera, were given refuge on Crete. Having weapons the warriors declared martial law in the face of the disaster and then they established Mycenaean rule on Crete.

NOTICING A DISJUNCTION BETWEEN IMAGE AND STORY

In contrast to the graceful and grace-filled images from Keph culture, the later historical Greek texts insist on a dark, violent story. The ancient Greeks told the myth of the Minotaur, a lurid tale which begins with a Queen's consummated passion for a bull which results in a monstrous progeny which feeds on the best of the young men and women of Athens until an Athenian prince aided by a Minoan priestess slays the monster.

No images of human sacrifice, superstition, violence, conflict, or war occur in Keph culture. There is no support in the art or artifacts of the Keph society on Crete for the tale of the bloody bull-monster or of a monstrous society.

The actual Keph scene is reflected in the ring seals of the cow and the bull. This is the scene of the gentle bull, a scene in which the power of wild nature, symbolized by the powerful adult bull, has been tamed, gentled, and even socialized to cooperate with humans, even in play. Such a bull may have been raised

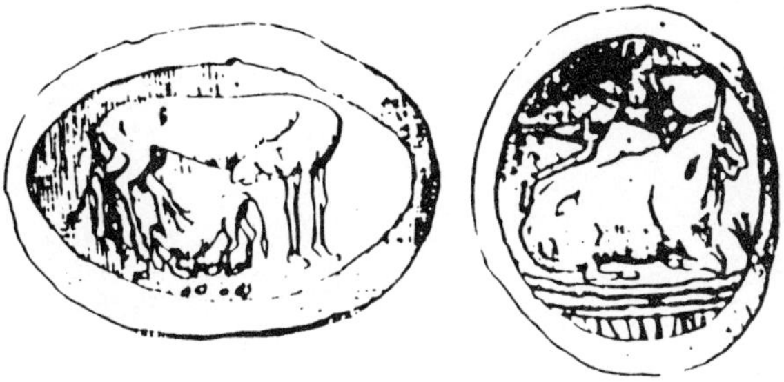

on a woman's lap, an image which resonates with human experience and also appears in Neolithic art in Anatolia. This bull has been trained to participate in the bull-leaping dance, a sport or ritual ceremony conducted at Knossos. Here we see the acrobat practicing with the quiet cooperation of the bull. The scene is that of cooperation between human and beast: there is no hint of opposition between human and nature here or elsewhere in Keph imagery.

The cow nursing and licking her calf, creating a circle or cycle of caring, illustrates the natural scene, or scene of nature, which is the scene of Keph culture. Such naturalistic Keph imagery superbly evokes the concept of culture in harmony with nature. Adjectives which can be applied to this pair of seals are the same ones which can be applied in general to

Keph culture -- harmonious, gracious, graceful, gentle, playful, light, enlightened, and at-one-with raw nature.

NOTICING IMAGES AS TEXT

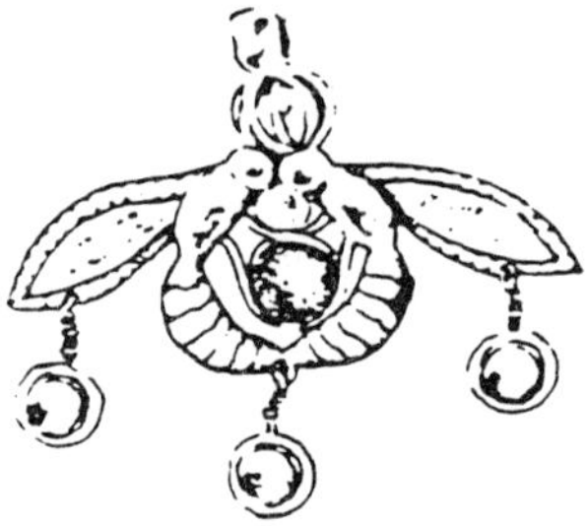

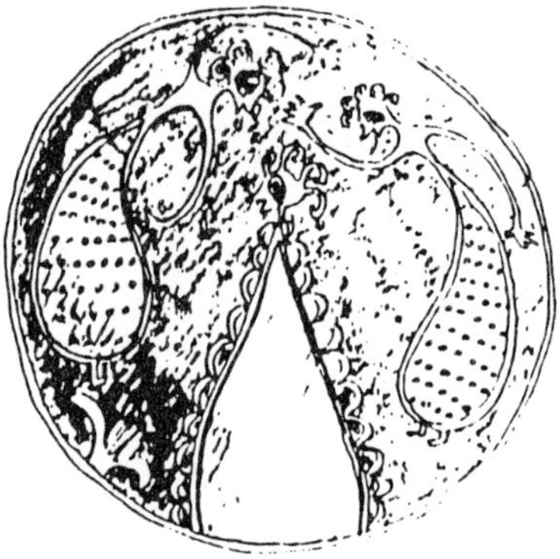

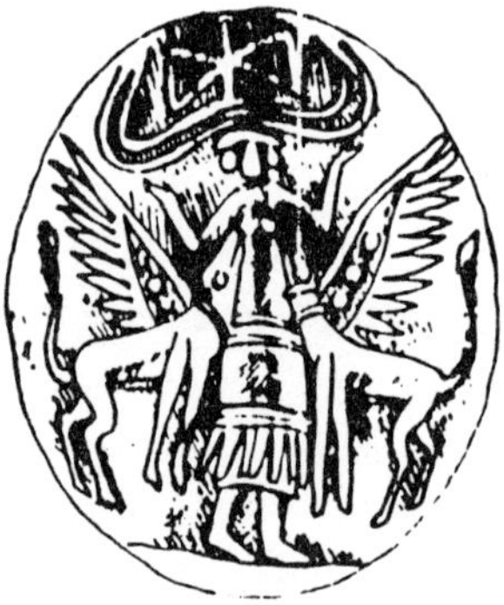

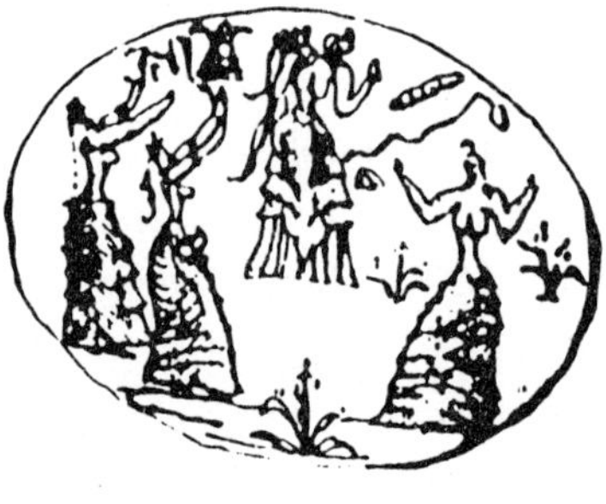

When images are taken seriously as text, patterns of images begin to emerge. For example all the bees in

Keph imagery call us to notice not only that bees were important, but that women took the part of bee characters in rituals, dance, and dramatic enactment. What the story was about can be inferred logically.

Logically the Keph people characterized their society as a bee-like society. The Keph people are illustrated with startlingly narrow, bee-like waists, which, once we notice the importance of bee imagery, signifies that these were the people of the "bee" culture. The flower motif then, so popular in Keph art, signifies the scene of flowers which is characteristically the scene of bees. In fact, the word "Keph" is etymologically linked to flowers and flowering in an array of usages, including the head, which is the seat of intellectual flowering; the birth image known as the "crowning," that moment during childbirth when the top of the head appears in the birth canal; and the hill mound, or archeological "tell" of Knossos, which was the seat of the birth and flowering of Keph culture.

In <u>Goddesses and Gods of Old Europe</u> Marija Gimbutas notes the bee imagery in "Old European" neolithic culture and links it forward in time to bee imagery in ancient Crete (pp. 181-190). Gaye Manifold, professor of drama at the University of La Verne, in an unpublished study, notes that the mythology of bees is embedded in modern natural histories of bees and links bee societies back in time to bee priestess societies in Greek antiquity at Ephesus, Delphi, and Eleusis. I note that the Keph culture of Crete interfaces a bee-identified, female-centered perspective between a matrifocal perspective evidenced in Old European neolithic imagery and a male-defined patriarchal perspective evident in Western traditions. The latter perspective is more than familiar to us, because although it originated in Greek antiquity most of us have assimilated the current operating version of male-defined culture from birth.

Through bee imagery Keph society expressed identification with the existential natural world of bees. By looking back and forth between the existential natural world of bees and Keph culture we can begin to uncover a storied relationship between Keph society and bee society which will serve to enrich our own perception of the history of human culture, which in turn will enrich our imagination about possible futures for human societies.

The existential beehive is more than female-centered. The source of all the progeny of the hive is the fertile female at its core. But again it is important to note that Keph imagery does not refer to the scene of birth or the scene of pregnancy, a frequently illustrated scene in neolithic cultures. In fact, Keph female images are seldom seen holding infants. There are, however, references to lactation, an image-text for the scene of nurture.

For bees the hive is the constructed center of the colony. Worker bees go out from and return to the central hive, some gathering pollen and some gathering nectar from blossoming earth. If the hive is successful it will continue for many years and also send forth new colonies which will construct new hives to be organically constructed to fit an ecologically favorable site.

The historical scene of Keph society very closely fits the ecological scene of bees. Knossos was the first settlement. It provided the resources and population for additional settlements on Crete. During the period of Keph florescence, centers such as Malia and

Phaistos were patterned after Knossos. Each was organically constructed to take advantage of scenes of natural beauty.

Keph society on Crete was organized around the main "hive," Knossos, which was the ceremonial center of the culture. The ceremonial life of Knossos appears to have been organized around a central female character, represented in one wall painting as a member of the Keph community, indistinguishable from any other individual in the community except that she was in the ceremonial position of receiving the gifts which others, both men and women, brought her. This central female character, conceptually equal to every other Keph person, appears to have been analagous to a centralizing divine female character who would logically be the numinous presence of place, the character which gave generously to the original settlers and all their progeny, the character honored by the placement of the sacred central "dancing court" at Knossos, and the character represented in image as the numinous female bee-character flanked by griffins, divine animal characters.

Bees "sing" and "dance" as they work and on occasions perform "ceremonial dances." The nuptial flight of the new queen with the fertile males might be identified, not as a sexual scene but nevertheless as an exuberant dance and the swarm of a new colony as another dance. These "ceremonial occasions" usually occur during the season of flowers, i.e., in springtime and summer. Dancing, accompanied by music and singing, is an important subject in Keph art. Bee dancers are women in bee costume who take the part of characters in the scene of flowers. These dancers logically celebrate the renewed and ever-renewing cycle of annual growth, ergo, the Keph people through ceremonial ritual intellectually acknowledged, with devotion and reverence, the existential character of the natural world.

NOTICING A FAMILIAR TEXT IN A DIFFERENT CONTEXT

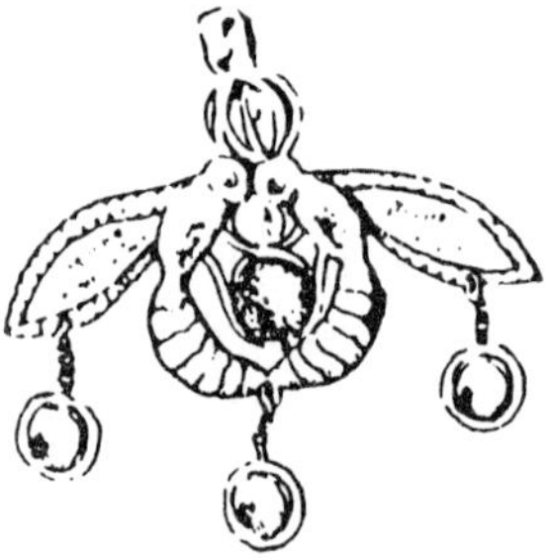

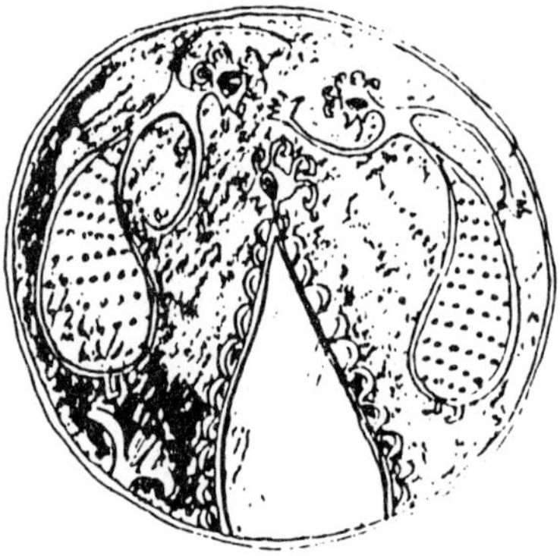

"As in heaven so on earth" is a familiar text which occurs frequently in the Old European imagery illustrated in Goddesses and Gods of Old Europe 7000-3500 B.C.: Myths, Legends and Cult Images by Gimbutas. Sometimes a female character is shown giving birth, sometimes a female character is illustrated as a double image, and sometimes a mirror image is used. In Egyptian and Hittite imagery contemporary with Keph society, a divine female character holds a mirror, which is reflecting the cosmos to the manifest world and reflecting the manifest world to the cosmic realm.

"As in heaven so on earth" is the image-text of the "dancing bees" plate and the honeybee pendant. The golden bee pendant is from the beginning of the period florescence around 2200 B.C. and the "dancing bees" plate from the middle period, around 1800 B.C.

The elegance of the bee pendant suggests a divine pair conceptualized as two aspects of one whole: it would be logical to read this image as the divine character of the shared social order to bees and Keph society. On another level, the gold of this pendant resonates with the golden honey of the beehive in the scene of natural abundance. It also suggests human culture constructed in harmony with raw nature, and culture dependent on nature.

The text of the "dancing bee" scene can also be read as a double image in which the central figure is analagous to the flower. The red female character emerging in this scene is substantial but numinous. She is logically the beneficent force of spring manifest in the pushing forth of spring flowers. The power of spring and her flowers activates the bees, sends humans out to tend shoots of the new crop in the field, releases human joy because the annual temperate zone crisis of winter is over, and arouses human enjoyment of flowers. She is also logically the divine presence which pushes Keph culture to flowering.

HOW IMAGES PUSH US TO SEE THROUGH TODAY'S TARNISHED SURFACE TOWARD SPIRIT-CENTERED WHOLENESS

These image-texts are seed texts, sprouting, growing, quivering to flower. As in the days when Zeus acknowledged the primacy of the cyclical processes of Demeter, we need to bring the world into harmony with ecology. In the words of Peggy Cleveland, we need to Mother the Earth. In the meantime, we can acknowledge the image-text of our own lives and imagine the world as we desire it to be.

> I am a "Protestant." My mother has never gone to church, my maternal grandmother occasionally went to church to "hear the music," my maternal great-grandmother took me by the hand and enrolled me in Christian Science Sunday School at the edge of my first memories, and I continued to go every Sunday until one Sunday when I was 16 and realized I was being pushed to choose between the material world and the spiritual world, between science and Christian Science, between the enjoyment of world and church dogma, and I never went to Sunday School again. Ever since, I have been searching the world for a model of spirit-centered wholeness to affirm my personal perception of wholeness. I have been disappointed by images. For example, the image of the moving yin and yang incorporated in the globe of Tao, so like the image of our Earth from space, looks correct, but it moves within a male-centered text, and therefore, it speaks to me by way of translation into my woman's experience.
>
> I am "white." My family laughed at my animated interest in the African drums played by the father of a black boy in my first year of school; they ignored my friendships with Jewish girls in high school: in these and many other ways my family taught me that "white" means superior and "color"

means other. Nevertheless, I have not been able to comprehend what difference color makes when it comes to death or suffering or love or enjoyment.

I imagine an enlightened and enlivening world in which human beings live in different societies, but everywhere live through a perspective of rootedness and connectedness and in a consciousness which nurtures their human birthright as spiritual and aesthetic beings, ergo, that all the people of the earth live within a global consciousness of psychic and social wholeness.

I am "middle-class." I have experienced my life in a hierarchy of privilege. I have been comfortable but watched the greater privilege of others with envy. I have been made aware of the wants of the others who are less privileged, so that when I am hurting I must discount my hurt because others hurt so much more, and then I hate them because my hurt is so great. I have also become aware that my privilege hurts others: that the privilege of others hurts me.

I am "Western." I have watched the bulldozers push over houses I have lived in and cover over the earth with asphalt where flowers grew. I have watched fruit trees ripped from the earth and houses planted in their place. I have watched machines scrape and gouge away blossoming plants and rippling sand and then stood by while faceless men planted factories, refineries, sewer "plants," and power "plants" on the wounded earth.

I have lived forty-nine years. I have lived in the scenes of weapons and violence all my life.

Since I can remember, and before, in the relative sanctuary of home and in the public streets, I have been struggling to accommodate the fear of unaccountable, violent attack at the hands of a shadowy boogey. I have looked within and without for that "boogey." I have looked through the archaeological archives of human history. The earliest uncovered scene of violence occurs on the horizon of civilization: the image marks the invention of the institution of war through which one people force another people, against their will and at the expense of some of their lives, to be subjugated: this first embodiment of the boogey of violent force is dated c. 3400 B.C. I notice that the scene of war is embodied in a man, a King. In contrast to this image are the images from the Keph civilization of Crete, images of open human grace, of culture moving in harmony with wild nature, of enspirited organic order, of animated play, and of aroused delighted enjoyment. I notice that these images are female-centered.

I am a woman. In the world, almost globally certainly in my world, I notice that I, as woman, embody the concept of other. However much I struggle against this unsubstantial notion, I meet it in the world and it stops me. I notice that this means that in some way beyond my comprehension the destructive energies of the world are considered to be my fault even though I am substantially barred from the public world which has the power to compose, arrange, engineer, and activate these destructive energies. I have lived for the most part in the isolation of the home, tied to the hearth, working on the periphery of the public world where I have done my best to help imagine and activate a different world. I notice that even what I have imagined has often been suggested to me by men: for most of my life men have also defined my most intimate experiences: all my life men have mediated all my actions in the public sphere and have thus far effectively stopped me. I have experienced most of life as fragmentation from my self, alienation from those with whom I have had my most intimate relationships, including my mother, my husband, and my children. I have felt powerless to change the world to protect those I love from undue harm or to protect the Earth from untoward harm. I notice that these experiences are usual among women.

I imagine that before I can fully reclaim my spirit, my wholeness, and my self, I must be empowered. I imagine that before I can be empowered the image of woman must substantially be incorporated into the definition of human in the world. I imagine that before the consciousness of the world can change substantially empowered women must be welcomed as fully conscious, active, and engaged participants in the world. I imagine that all these changes are linked to the image of "god" in the world: it may be that Our Mother is the moving principle of life on Earth and that She enacts authentic spirit-centered wholeness: it is logical that Our Mother animates and brings forth the world with its allure of intelligence and its delightful variety. I imagine that Our Mother, the Mother of all living, must be fully met, for life on Earth to continue.

Footnote

[1] These drawings were made by artist Ebet Dudley from archeological material in the catalog of the Museum at Heraklion.

References

Gimbutas, Marija. Goddesses and Gods of Old Europe 7000-3500 B.C.: Myths, Legends, and Cult Images. Los Angeles: University of California Press, revised 1980.

Griffin, Susan. Woman and Nature: The Roaring Inside Her. New York: Harper and Row, 1978.

Mellaart, James. The Neolithic of the Near East. New York: Charles Scribner's Sons, 1975.

PSYCHOLOGICAL WHOLENESS

Wholeness: The Perspectives of Indian Idealism

John E. Roberts

The Central Task

This paper sets as its primary task the definition of "Spirit," "spirit," and "wholeness" in the context of "spirit-centered wholeness" and approaches that task from the perspective of Vedic philosophy. Specific attention is focused on the historical Advaita Vedanta of Sri Shankara and the contemporary expression of Vedic philosophy in the writings and applied teachings of Paramahansa Yogananda. Paramahansa Yogananda is perhaps best known as the founder of Self-Realization Fellowship/Yogoda Satsanga Society of India (SRF/YSS).

A secondary task of this paper is to elaborate the absolute necessity for the recognition of the need to structure any definitional and operational activities of the type undertaken by the IRW1 upon the foundation of a well-articulated philosophical position.

The disciple-perspective from which this paper is written is that of psychology and philosophy. These disciplines are viewed as necessarily compatible in that philosophy establishes the conceptual-theoretical foundation and psychology provides the conceptual-specific and applicational foci.

Problem Statement

There is in the disseminate literature of the IRW a clear, intentional, and pervasive concern directed toward the need to identify and define those numerous and complex interfaces between the many peoples of the planet (including their established institutions of religion, government, science, education, agriculture, law, art, psychology, medicine, etc.), the biosphere, and God--the Universal Creator. Equally compelling is the Institute's impetus to effect a corpus of unified knowledge and wisdom replete with correlate prescriptions for effective cross-discipline dialog, information exchange, etc. In addition there are prescriptive criteria for salugenic practices and beliefs; androgenous approaches and attitudes.

All factors considered, the natural and logical first question to arise is: "What, if anything, does each and every human being, every animate and inanimate object in creation, and God actually have in common or at the very least share"? The need for there to be such a "thing" is strongly felt or intuited within each serious and sincere-minded person who, for whatever reason, seeks an answer to the "unification" problem. Further, a successful analytic quest for this nuclear sine qua non must in some indisputable way be perceived as the primigenial necessary and sufficient condition for any acceptable synthesis resultants.

We can seriously and legitimately ask if there is in fact such a common element of the type required because, while the belief may be strongly intuited, the fact remains that science has not found an acceptable answer. And if empirical evidence of immanent proof is not extant, we who are educated and enculturated in the

Western scientific-intellectual tradition quite naturally tend to doubt the possibility of any such existence. In fact the Cartesian-mechanistic-reductionistic tradition which still predominates and drives most scientific and academic endeavors virtually precludes such a hypothesis/discovery possibility. The thesis that this tradition is no longer tenable is compellingly supported by an exponentially increasing body. The quest for a vital and creative approach thus appears a prime necessity.

The Need for a Comprehensive Philosophy

A central thesis of this paper is that any serious attempt to define "Spirit-centered wholeness" must of necessity invoke a philosophical position. It is held that this necessity will obtain whether any definitional attempt deliberately invokes and makes public its philosophical position or instead chooses consciously or unconsciously to remain mute on the subject. This position is held as incontrovertible.

Any philosophical system capable of meeting the rigorous IRW challenge must be sufficiently well developed, articulated, coherent, and testable logically and pragmatically so as to meet the universal needs of all who apply. Several major problems inhere in our philosophical quest however; one intrinsic in Western philosophy, one encompassing Eastern philosophy. A brief look at each of these problems illuminates their respective natures.

A Central Problem in Western Philosophy

Western philosophy for some time now has been in an apparent state of deterioration. This is avowed not only by scientists, professionals, and laymen but by philosophers themselves. One reason for this decline is the charge that Western philosophy has become impotent and as a result has failed to issue in any theories about the nature of reality. Viewing this problem from the perspective of psychology and through the perceptions of two philosophers, let us consider several examples. First, the testimony of Armstrong (1968):

> When we consider modern philosophers who write about the mind, it is often difficult to determine just how their view of time fits into the classification offered. This might be taken to be a criticism of the classification, but in fact I do not think that it should be so taken. I believe there are two other reasons why it is so hard to place their views. In the first place, there is no doubt that the question of the nature of the mind is one of the utmost difficulty. When we add this to the tentative and piecemeal character of a great deal of modern philosophizing, it is not surprising that many philosophers have simply not come to a clear decision about their view of the mind.
>
> There is, however, what I think is a much darker and less intellectually honourable reason for the difficulty that there often is in discovering their view. Since the work of Wittgenstein, it has been fashionable to maintain that philosophy does not issue in any theories at all about the nature of reality. Hence it is not the <u>business</u> of the philosopher to maintain any theory of mind. I think that this doctrine has proved intellectually corrupting, for in fact it

> is quite impossible to be in such a theory-free state if you think at all extensively on philosophical topics. Those philosophers who believe that they are in such a theory-free state are really being moved by obscure and ill-formulated theories which escape any criticism or correction because they are never brought out into the open where they can be clearly considered.

There is a second major problem area in Western philosophy and that centers on philosophical methodology and the scope of problem focus; both of which have succeeded in producing "bad images." Campbell (1970) explains:

> The Mind-Body problem . . .illustrates the relationship between philosophy and other intellectual pursuits, notably in natural science. Philosophy has sometimes fallen into disrepute among sensible men because this relationship has been distorted or misunderstood. The old bad image of philosophy is of an arrogant and foolish armchair dogmatism. Philosophers are seen as proclaiming doctrines as "proven by pure reason" in wanton disregard of what hard experimental and theoretical work might discover. Such a harsh view of philosophy is not dissipated by the spectacle of Aristotle "proving" that the planets move in circles; Descartes rejecting even the possibility of empty space, and Kant arguing that there can be no indeterminacy in physics.
>
> Philosophy's new bad image -- mini-philosophy -- is one of pedantic triviality. The new distortion affirms that philosophy's concern is solely with bringing to light the content of the concepts men use in their thought about the world.

> Philosophy is a modest inquiry into the meanings of words and the implications of sentences, and cannot determine truth or falsehood. This view of philosophy as impotent, as no more significant than butterfly collecting, has complex causes in the despair of twentieth-century intellectuals. It has given its most characteristic expression in the thought of Wittgenstein, who said, for example, "Philosophy leaves everything as it is."

We shall leave the problem of Western philosophy at this point with the tacit understanding that the problems cited are sufficient to suggest that this discipline will not serve the needs of the task. Let us turn next to an examination of Eastern philosophy.

<u>A Problem Encompassing Eastern Philosophy</u>

Let it be stated at the onset that the field of Eastern philosophy is enormously wide in scope and that it is not the intention of this paper to engage in any kind of survey activity. The task here is simply to focus on one philosophy with the choice being Vedic, the philosophy of orthodox Hinduism.

Perhaps the single most outstanding problem surrounding Vedic philosophy is the paucity of knowledge and the resultant dearth of understanding which pervades most people's minds on the subject. Dasgupta, one of the world's outstanding scholars in Indian philosophy, has stated that "the achievements of the ancient Indians in the field of philosophy are but very imperfectly known to the world at large, and it is unfortunate that the condition is not better even in India" (1932, p. 1). This problem spawns even greater problems when people imbued with partial and faulty knowledge become the "authorities" on the subject and render inappropriate judgements and dispense false teachings. As Dasgupta phrases it: "Much harm has already been done by the circulation of opinions that the culture and philosophy of India was dreamy and abstract" (1932, p. vii). Taimni offers a more detailed picture of the problem as it pertains to Yoga philosophy (one of the six philosophical systems in the Vedic tradition):

> The philosophy _Yoga_ deals with some of the greatest mysteries of life and the Universe and so it must inevitably be associated with an atmosphere of profound mystery . . . . some teachers of _Yoga_ have attempted to meet this difficulty by taking out of the philosophy and technique of _Yoga_ those particular practices which are easy to understand and pratice, placing these before the general public as _Yogic_ teachings. Many of these practices like _Asana_ . . . . etc. [seem to be] of a purely physical nature and when divorced from the higher and essential teachings of _Yoga_ reduce their systems to a science of physical culture on a par with other systems of a similar nature. This over-simplification of the problem of _Yogic_ life, though it has done some good and helped some people to live a saner and healthier physical life, has greatly vulgarized the movement for _Yogic_ culture and produced a wrong impression, especially in the West, about the real purpose and technique of _Yoga_. (1971, pp. v-vi)

If the problem is as pervasive as it has been rendered, one could appropriately wonder if there is a viable solution. Clearly the philosophy has been and is known by certain individuals, so it is not intended that one should wrongfully conclude that it is not knowable. The problem basically resides in the general lack of understanding and the pervasive misunderstanding.

The solution proposed by this paper, relative to the IRW definitional task, is to bring to awareness for consideration, the Vedic commentaries and teachings of Sri Shankara and the contemporary East-West expositions on Vedic philosophy as contained in the philosophy and teachings of Paramahansa Yogananda.

Why Consider Vedic Philosophy as a Viable Response to the Call to Define "Spirit-Centered Wholeness"?

The immanent import of Indian philosophy has long been recognized by both East and West. Dasgupta sheds immediate light on its potential relevance to contemporary issues and problems:

> Most of the problems that are still debated in modern philosophical thought occurred in more or less divergent forms to the philosophers of India. Their discussions, difficulties and solutions when properly grasped in connection with the problems of our own times may throw light on the course of the process of the future reconstruction of modern thought. The discovery of the important features of Indian philosophical thought, and a due appreciation of their full significance, may turn out to be as important to modern philosophy as the discovery of Sanskrit has been to the investigation of modern philological researches. (1932, p. viii)

Let us consider further the views of Cousin and Schlegel as representatives of Western recognition:

The French historian, Victor Cousin, said:

> When we read with attention the philosophical monuments of the Orient--above all, those of India--we discover there many a truth so profound . . . that we are constrained to bend the knee before the philosophy of the East, and to see in this cradle of the human race the native land of the highest philosophy." Schlegel observed: "Even the loftiest philosophy of the Europeans, the idealism of reason as set forth by the Greek philosophers, appears--in comparison with the abundant life and vigor of Oriental idealism--like a feeble Promethean spark against the full flood of sunlight. (Cited in Yogananda, 1979, p. 86)

Vedic philosophy is a philosophy of idealism. The essential significance of this fact lies in the understanding that "idealism" is herein taken to mean that there is but one reality which is spiritual in its nature and all things are explainable as existing in and through it. Vedic idealism holds this reality to be Spirit-God.

If Vedic idealism can be accepted as meaning that there is <u>only</u> Spirit and that all other things can be meaningfully and relevantly described as existing in and through Spirit, then examination of this philosophy is viewed as being of paramount value in service to the avowed task.

Prospective

Attention will next be directed to the subject of Vedic philosophy from an historical perspective together with a very brief introduction to the central tenets. The Vedanta philosophy of Sri Shankara is also presented in the section.

The second section to follow presents the philosophy and teachings of Paramahansa Yogananda which includes a brief recapitulation of the historical foundations and a summary of the central doctrinal elements. The principal focus of this section, however, is directed to an explication of the ontology of creation with attention also directed on the human being.

The final section of this paper reviews central primary and secondary tasks, recapitulates certain salient features, postulates synthesis resultants, and renders the definitions for which this task was primarily initiated; viz., "Spirit," "spirit," "wholeness," and "Spirit-centered wholeness."

Exposition will progress using the developmental approach; meaning simply the contents of one section serve as a basis for the next. A task of such scope can, at best, be only summary in nature and, hence, do little more than suggest a "pointing of the way."

VEDIC PHILOSOPHY -- AN OVERVIEW

Introduction

When the term "Vedic" philosophy is used, it is traditionally taken to mean that philosophy as contained in the Vedas (Samhitas, Aranyakas, Brahmanas, and the Upanishads) and the six derivative orthodox philosophical systems (Nyaya, Vaisesika, Yoga, Sankhya, Mimamsa, and Vedanta). The six orthodox systems are so named because they each appeal to the incontestable scriptural authority embodied in the Vedas. By contrast, the heterodox schools of Indian philosophy (Buddhist, Jaina, Carvaka, etc.) do not endeavor to establish their validity on Vedic authority.

Two interesting and important considerations revolve around any serious endeavor to understand the import of the Vedas, viz., their origin and age. The Vedas were considered, and remain so to this day, embodiments of the highest knowledge revealed by God to humankind, they are thus considered infallible and, as such, they are the sacred incontestable scriptures of Hinduism. Dasgupta (1932) discusses these two considerations:

> It is indeed difficult to say when the earliest portions of these compositions came into existence. Many shrewd guesses have been offered, but none of them can be proved to be incontestably true. Max Muller supposed the date to be 1200 B.C., Haug 2400 B.C. and Bal Gangadhar Tilak 4000 B.C. The ancient Hindus seldom kept any historical record of their literary, religious or political achievements. The Vedas were handed down from mouth to mouth from a period of unknown antiquity, and the Hindus generally believed that they were never composed by men. It was therefore generally supposed that either they were taught by God to the sages, or that they were of themselves revealed to the sages who were the "seers" (*mantradrasta*) of the hymns. Thus we find that when some time had elapsed after composition of the Vedas, people had come to look upon them not only as very old, but so old that they had, theoretically at least, no beginning in time, though they were believed to have been revealed at some unknown remote period at the beginning of each creation. (p. 10)

The revelatory occurrences which ultimately culminated in the Vedas produced an interesting problem.

The process, being experiential and not theoretical or speculative in nature, and the essentially verbatim chronicling of the results, resulted in a body of works almost totally lacking in systemic structure. It was this outcome which prompted the need for systematic disentanglement of the wisdom-threads woven throughout the Vedas. The result was the evolution of the six systems of orthodox Hindu philosophy.

Central Tenets

Scholars, in their efforts to understand more successfully the Vedas, have long and earnestly struggled to identify the nuclear elements. In his attempts to distill out any systemic semblance, Duessen (1966) concluded he could reasonably and confidently postulate four divisions within the Upanishads:

I. Theology: the doctrine of Brahman (God) as the first principle of all things.

II. Cosmology: the doctrine of the evolution of this principle to form the universe.

III. Psychology: the doctrine of the entrance of Brahman as Soul [Atman] into the universe evolved from Him.

IV. Eschatology and Ethics: the doctrine of the fate of the soul after death, and the manner of life which is therefore required. (p. 52)

These four divisions succinctly demonstrate that the fundamental philosophical teaching of the Veda is that of monism and idealism. Hiriyanna (1973) elaborates this observation:

> The prevailing view in them [the Upanishads] is monistic and absolutistic. That is to say, they teach the ultimate reality is one and only

> one . . . . The teaching is also idealistic in the sense that the single reality is conceived of as spiritual in its nature and that everything else is explained as existing in and through it . . . . This is not to say that either pluralism or the belief that the ultimate entities are many, and realism or the belief that matter is as real as spirit or mind, are unknown to the Upanishads, taken as a whole. It only means that . . . they are not conspicuous in them. (p. 19)

To summarize, the universal doctrine of Vedic philosophy resolves to the equation: God (Brahman) = Soul (Atman). Duessen (1966) explains:

> That is to say--the Brahman, the power which presents itself to us materialized in all existing things, which creates, sustains, preserves, and received back into itself again all worlds, this eternal infinite divine power is again all worlds, this eternal infinite divine power is identical with Atman, with that which, after stripping off everything external, we discover in ourselves as our real most essential being, our individual self, the soul. This identity of the Brahman and the Atman, of God and the soul is the fundamental thought of the entire doctrine of the Upanishads.

It is upon the cornerstone of this seminal fact, viz., God-Soul, the "Spirit-centered wholeness" is to be defined in this paper.

The Vedic Philosopher

There is one concluding point requiring presentation before leaving this section. This point is essential not only to a proper understanding of Vedic philosophy from an applied dimension, but it is also of cardinal importance in this definitional task for the IRW. The subject pertains to the Vedic philosophers themselves.

The absolute and ultimate avowed goal in Indian philosophy is the conscious reuniting of the individual soul with God. This goal is termed moksha or liberation; meaning liberation from the pain born of the soul's ignorance of its true nature. When this liberation is achieved, it signifies the culmination of the highest knowledge; it is the consummate act of enlightenment--Self-realization. Hiriyanna (1973) offers a disclosing statement on the manner of life exercised by these philosophers and, importantly, brings the vital link between philosophy and religion into awareness:

> This enlightenment, however, does not mean only an intellectual apprehension of the view that all is one, but also an actual realization of that unity in our own experience. In other words, the aim of studying philosophy is not merely to gratify theoretical curiosity, however disinterested that curiosity may be; it is also to live the right kind of life, consequently adjusting one's conduct to one's intellectual convictions. It is in this sense of devotion to worthier living and not in the sense of dogma or superstition, that religion is blended with philosophy in India. (pp. 15-16)

Prabhavananda (1974) amplifies this perspective by further rendering the essential nature of the true philosopher:

> The prophetic souls who, with a noble passion for truth, strive hard to understand the mystery

of the world and give utterance to it, spending laborious days and sleepless nights, are philosophers in a vital sense of the term.

Indian philosophy is thus not a mere way of thinking but a way of life, a way of light, and a way of truth. To become a philosopher is to become transformed in life, renewed in mind, and baptized in spirit. (p. 16)

From the foregoing, another essential feature of Indian philosophy thus stands revealed -- the individual philosopher. This individual we see as one who with profound dedication, aspires to a higher knowledge while simultaneously laboring to quicken the latent and immanent truth in that knowledge through the agency of purposeful action. It is in this context that we catch the glimmer of a germinal light regarding the nature of "wholeness," e.g., "to become transformed in life, renewed in mind, and baptized in spirit."

The Philosophy of Sri Shankara

It was stated earlier that the Upanishads are part of the Vedas and that the philosophy of Vedanta is one of the six philosophical systems of Vedic philosophy. We find an interesting connection here in that "Vedanta" means literally "end of the Vedas" (Veda-anta) and the Upanishads are the end of the Vedas). Therefore the Vedanta philosophy is that system predicated on the teaching of the Upanishads. The Upanishads were also stated to embody the distillate knowledge of all the Vedas. The principal formulator of the Vedanta system is the philosopher-seer Badarayana. Sri Shankara was the principal commentator on Badarayana's monism.

Yogananda (1979) has referred to Sri Shankara as "India's greatest philosopher." He writes:

> Lord Shankara was a rare combination of saint, scholar, and man of action. Though he lived only thirty-two years, many of them were spent in arduous travel to every part of India, spreading his advaita doctrine. Millions gathered eagerly to hear the solacing flow of wisdom from the lips of the barefoot man.
>
> Shankara's reforming zeal included the reorganization of the ancient monastic Swami Order. He also founded four maths (monastic educational centers) . . . . The four maths of the great monist . . . gave free instruction in Sanskrit grammar, logic and Vedanta philosophy. (p. 110)

In another statement, Yogananda (1976) comments that Shankara "expounded God not as a negative abstraction, but as positive, eternal omnipresent, ever-new Bliss" (p. 480).

The philosophical position advanced by Sri Shankara is properly known as Advaita Vedanta, the qualifier "Advaita" denoting a non-dual, strictly monistic teaching. In defining his position, and articulating its principal goal, Yogananda (1976) writes: "Vedanta declares that God is the only reality and that creation is essentially an illusion. As man is the only creature capable of conceiving God, man must himself be divine, and his duty therefore is to realize his true nature." (1976, pp. 482-3)

Sri Shankara set down a dual epistemological position characterized by a higher and a lower knowledge. The lower knowledge is viewed as relative in that it functions within phenomenal creation so it is therefore realistic in its philosophical orientation. The higher knowledge is concerned only with the Noumenon, the transcendental Self, and is consequently absolute, monistic, and idealistic in nature. Both knowledge types are considered essential in the attainment of Self-realization, the goal of all life.

In summary, the quintessential teaching in the Advaita Vedanta of Sri Shankara is that God alone exists, all souls are a part of God and are therefore the same in essence as God. The principal problem of existence centers on individual ignorance; viz., that obfuscating power which veils each soul in creation and thus precludes the direct experience (hence the ultimate knowing) of its true nature--divinity itself. The central epistemological thrust of Advaita Vedanta consequently addresses the need for right knowledge and asserts that the highest knowledge is that which, when coupled with right action, dispels individual ignorance. The consummate attainment of ultimate knowledge is referred to as Self-realization where the capitalization of "Self" denotes the soul in contradistinction to the lower-case "self" which signifies the ego-identified consciousness.

We proceed next to the philosophy and teachings of Paramahansa Yogananda and in so doing are introduced to the cosmological and ontological doctrines subsumed under the mantle of Vedic philosophy. And, of significant importance, in this next section we will also be introduced to certain applicational considerations which, as previously indicated, constitute the "other half" of Vedic philosophy.

THE PHILOSOPHY AND TEACHINGS OF PARAMAHANSA YOGANANDA

Introduction

Yogananda's avowed mission was not formally to

explicate Vedic philosophy in any scholarly sense; it was to present the necessary and sufficient knowledge and practices essential to enable an individual to achieve Self-realization. As he once stated: "I came not to preach a doctrine; I came to teach a living truth." Yogananda expressly chose to avoid the use of Sanskrit words in his writings to the extent possible. Accordingly, many formal philosophical terms are not in evidence per se; the principles, however, clearly are. This subject is brought to attention simply to point out that if one is interested in overlaying the template of Yogananda's teachings to determine correspondence, it can be efficiently done, but one will need to know and understand Vedic philosophy to some extent to do so.

Yogananda (1976) has defined Self-realization as: "The knowing--in body, mind, and soul--that we are one with the omnipresence of God; that we do not have to pray that it come to us, that we are not merely near it at all times, but that God's omnipresence is our omnipresence; that we are just as much a part of Him now as we ever will be. All we have to do is improve our knowing." (p. 480). Yogananda (1976) also defines "Self" as "individualized Spirit [the soul], whose nature is ever-existing, ever-conscious, ever-new joy . . . . The soul is the true and immortal nature of man, and of all living forms of life" (pp. 480-81).

Immanent Vedic Doctrine

Three systems of Vedic philosophy are in outstanding evidence in the philosophy and teachings of Paramahansa Yogananda: Sankhya, Vedanta, and Yoga. For present purposes, the philosophy of Vedanta is considered sufficiently covered but it must always be remembered that in a very vital sense it constitutes the philosophical foundation upon which the principles of the other two systems depend. Consequently, only the systems of Sankhya and Yoga will be reviewed in this section.

The Sankhya System

The Sankhya cosmology has been recognized as a very complicated and difficult doctrine to understand. The dominant province of the Sankhya system is the explication of the Vedic cosmological doctrine. Both the Yoga and the Vedanta systems fundamentally rely on the Sankhya doctrine to explain the origin and nature of creation, and the process by which it evolves and is sustained.

The presence of the Sankhya doctrine in the philosophy of Paramahansa Yogananda is unambiguous; it is evidenced throughout his teachings. On occasion explicit reference to the subject is made; for example, in his forward to Sri Yukteswar's The Holy Science, he writes:

> It is owing to . . . Sri Yukteswar's unerring spiritual insight that it now becomes possible, through this book, to establish a fundamental harmony between the difficult biblical chapter Revelation and the Sankhya philosophy of India. (Yukteswar, 1972, pp. iii-iv)

Paramahansa Yogananda and his Guru, Swami Sri Yukteswar, have rendered the previously abstract doctrine far more intelligible to the modern scientific mind through the application of the concepts of magnetism, electricity, energy, etc.

It is one thing to say that all creation is evolved from the mind of God, but the knowing of how it occurs has immense importance for humankind. For it is in the knowing of these principles that the true science of human relations, the wellness of all living things, and the nature of physical causality, of mind, and of body is possible.

An introduction into how creation evolves from the mind of God is important to know and it further serves our avowed definition task. In the following statement, Yogananda (1976) provides this introduction. we will also observe in his statement the presence of Shankara's postulate of the higher and lower knowledge.

> Matter can be considered as not existing; but matter does have relative existence. Matter exists in relation to our mind and as an expression of invisible electronic forces that do exist, being unchangeable and immortal.
>
> Both water and ice are manifestations of invisible gases and have only formal transitory existence. Similarly, both mortal mind and matter are fleeting manifestations of Divine Consciousness, and possess merely formal existence; in reality only Cosmic Mind exists.
>
> Just as a child is born through the instrumentality of parents, so matter is dependent on mind for its existence. Matter is both from Divine Mind and is perceptible to moral mind; in itself and of itself, matter has no reality, no intrinsic existence.
>
> The blind or nonintellectual electronic forces of creation are nevertheless creative teleological agents because they contain within themselves the vibrations of the universal, conscious-of-itself life force or prana, which in turn issued from the fiat of Divinity.

> "God said let there be light: and there was light," [Genesis 1:3] that is, the projection of Divine Thought and Will became light or vibratory energy, the flowing forth of life current and electrons, which further vibrated more strongly and became the diverse subtle or unseen forces of nature, which in turn externalized themselves as the ninety-two principal elements of matter that constitute the universe. (1976, p. 57)

Yogananda, at another time, explained the process similarly but the subtle differences in rendering serve to resolve certain apparent perennial distinctions. In this statement we also have an explicit statement on the creation of the human being.

> The only difference between consciousness and matter, mind and body, is rate of vibration. Vibration is the motion of energy. How did this motion originate from the Cosmic Intelligence? All the vibrations in the ether are manifestations of the Intelligence-guided cosmic energy. Spirit as the unmanifested Absolute is without vibration or motion. Spirit manifested as the Creator is God the Father. The Creator first stirred His still Spirit with the motion of thoughts; thus God the Father's first projection of Creation was cosmic intelligent motion or vibrations of thought. This motion became stronger and grosser until it changed outwardly and manifested as cosmic light and cosmic sound (registered in the human body as the visible spiritual eye and the audible cosmic sound of <u>Aum</u> or <u>Amen</u>). The vibration of the conscious cosmic energy became progressively more gross, until it began to manifest as divine, semi-intelligent, instinctively

> guided electronic energy, and finally as the still grosser forms of gaseous, liquid, and solid energy.
>
> Likewise, the microcosm, or body of man, became into being first as a vibratory thought-form, the causal body. This in turn produced the grosser vibrations that make up the astral or energy body of man, which produces the still grosser vibrations that structure the solid physical body. Just as man uses electrically projected light and shadows on a movie screen, so the Cosmic Operator combines various thought-frozen vibrations of cosmic light and energy to produce in man's consciousness the "picture" of a solid physical body (1976, pp. 366-7).

What is perhaps most important to derive from the antecedent discussion is the awareness of the absolute interconnectedness of all creation, all life, all humanity. If we could but truly know and understand this intrinsic fundamental unity, and behave in harmony with that understanding, we would be able to (and want to) affect a greater appreciation for, and a sincere respect for, all elements of creation, all living things, and seek to promote a positive and loving relationship with each; and each with the other.

The Yoga System

Yogananda indicates that the word "Yoga" is from the Sanskrit yuj meaning "union." He states "The highest connotation of the word yoga in Hindu philosophy is union of the individual soul with Spirit through scientific methods of meditation" (1976, p. 483). In a pragmatic context, Yoga is known as the system which identifies and prescribes the various means by which the individual soul is able to achieve union with Spirit.

There are basically seven major yoga methods. The method taught by Paramahansa Yogananda is known as Raja Yoga. "Raja" means the "royal" (complete) yoga. Yogananda identifies it as the highest path to God-union and further states:

> It teaches scientific meditation as the ultimate means for realizing God, and includes the highest essentials from all other forms of Yoga. The Self-realization Fellowship Raja Yoga teachings outline a way of life leading to perfect unfoldment in body, mind, and soul, based on the foundation of Kriya Yoga meditation. (1976, p. 478)

Explaining Kriya Yoga, Yogananda states:

> The Sanskrit root of kriya is kri to do, to act and react; the same root is found in the word karma, the natural principle of cause and effect. Kriya Yoga is thus "union (yoga) with the Infinite through a certain action or rite (kriya)." (1976, p. 474)

Yogananda confirms that Patanjali was the foremost exponent of Yoga. And he is the acknowledged founder of the Yoga system of Indian philosophy. Patanjali outlined in his Yoga Sutras the principles of the yogic path, and presented them as eight steps. Yogananda (1979) identifies the eight steps:

> The first steps are (1) yama (moral conduct), and (2) niyama (religious observances). Yama is fulfilled by noninjury to others, truthfulness, nonstealing, continence, and noncovetousness. The niyama prescripts are purity of body and mind, contentment in all circumstances, self-discipline,

> self-study (contemplation), and devotion to God and guru.
>
> The next steps are (3) asana (right posture); the spinal column must be held straight, and the body firm in a comfortable position for meditation; (4) pranayama (control of prana, subtle life currents); and (5) pratyahara (withdrawal of the senses from external objects).
>
> The last steps are forms of yoga proper: (6) dharana (concentration), holding the mind to one thought; (7) dhyana (meditation); and (8) samadhi (superconscious experience). This Eightfold Path of Yoga leads to the final goal of Kaivalya (Absoluteness), in which the yogi realizes the Truth beyond all intellectual apprehension. (pp. 262-263)

In reviewing the preceding definitional statement on Yoga we can immediately identify the conjoint requirement for right thought and right action. In addition we see the distinction between the higher and the lower knowledge; the oneness of God and the goal of all life -- for the soul to reestablish its divine identity.

In summary, three Vedic systems have been identified as immanent in the philosophy and teachings of Paramahansa Yogananda. Emphasis was focused on a very brief sketch of the Sankhya and Yoga systems. The Sankhya system was shown to articulate the cosmological doctrine; Yoga the ethics, and the applicational principles necessary and sufficient to achieve Self-realization. The Vedanta system was acknowledged as the "foundation" philosophy. As such, it embodies the primary doctrines.

It is important here to mention again that Yogananda intended his teachings to emphasize the applied ("how-to") approach. But the knowledge of the "what" and the "why" is always present in support of the "how-to." It is in this context that the balancing of right knowledge with right action, as exemplified by the Vedic philosophers, is in evidence.

This concludes our overview of the philosophy and teachings of Paramahansa Yogananda. In the next, and last, section of this paper a summary of the principle tenets of Vedic philosophy, as set down in this paper, will be recapitulated; the derived elements synthesized to form the target definitions; and a review of the need for a declared philosophy position will be reviewed and repostulated.

SUMMARY AND CONCLUSION

This paper, at the outset, established a dual task. The assigned task was to define "Spirit-centered wholeness" from a discipline perspective. The second task, an assumed one, was to elaborate the absolute necessity for the recognition of the need to structure any definitional and operational activities of the type undertaken by the IRW upon the foundation of a well-articulated philosophical position. These two tasks will now be reviewed and addressed.

<u>"Spirit-Centered Wholeness" Defined</u>

The dual-discipline perspective from which this paper was developed was that of psychology and philosophy. The definition task was pursued from the perspective of Vedic philosophy which was basically identified as an idealistic, monistic, and absolutistic philosophy. The focus of the investigation was on the Vedic expressions as rendered in the Vedanta philosophy of Sri Shankara and the Self-Realization Fellowship of Paramahansa Yogananda. In the course of summarizing the philososphy and the central tenets, definitions of a direct and relevant nature arose.

Yogananda defined the "Self" (soul) as "individualized Spirit, whose nature is ever-existing, ever-conscious, ever-new joy." In this and a similar context we see the word "Spirit" used as synonymous with "God." And "Self" is used as a substitute for "soul" or "individualized Spirit," i.e., a manifested part of God. Examples of the qualities and descriptions of God's nature are also found as: "ever-existing, ever-conscious, ever-new joy." It is logically correct that this same nature is ascribed to the soul; the part should naturally manifest the same nature as that of which it is a part.

When the word "self" is used (i.e., not capitalized) it signifies the ordinary self which is taken to mean the ego or the personality of the mortal person. There is an important consideration regarding the self as ego which can be briefly touched on at this point. In Vedic doctrine the ego-principle is termed "ahankara" which literally translates as "I do." Yogananda defines this principle as the root cause of dualism or the seeming separation of man and his Creator." He goes on to note that: "by banishing ego-consciousness, man awakens to his divine identity, his oneness with the Sole Life: God" (Yogananda, 1976, p. 472).

The idea of "wholeness" in the context of the antecedent definitions has to be viewed as necessarily entailing the eradication of dualism and thereby establishing the unification of the part with the whole (the soul with God). This concept of the establishment of wholeness is, of course, the core teaching of Vedic philosophy and could correctly be said, philosophically speaking, to manifest the idealistic concept of wholeness.

Another definition of "wholeness" has been articulated by Howard Clinebell. His definition is: "'Wholeness' . . . means whole-person growth (physiological, intellectual, affective, interpersonal, spiritual) in a growth-nurturing social context (families, groups, institutions)." In the context of this paper, Clinebell's definition would have to be viewed as being within the purview of philosophical realism. This is an equally vital position for while it may not have been made clear before, it is a metaphysical truth that one must act in concert with the cosmic law as it operates in creation before one can transcend it. This position is thus a functional expression of the lower knowledge as expressed in Sri Shankara's epistemological doctrine.

The Need for a Philosophy

Clearly a true knowledge of the nature of the entities involved and of the spiritual laws governing the relations between such entities will serve to establish and perpetuate peace, understanding, compassion, forgiveness, and love between all and within each. Obviously an exploration of what this entails is beyond the limits of a paper such as this. This is not to beg the issue; rather it is to underscore the need for a guiding philosophy.

What is important to see from the foregoing is that given a philosophy of sufficient depth and breadth and one which embodies the principles of universal truth, the prescriptive principles inherent can be applied to in manifold manner. From these principles, discrete applicational prescriptives can be subsequently derived and implemented.

It has hopefully been sufficiently suggested and demonstrated that a viable philosophy is an absolute necessity for the task of defining "Spirit-centered wholeness."

Footnote

[1] IRW is an acronym for the Institute for Religion and Wholeness.

References

Armstrong, D. M. A Materialist Theory of Mind. London: Routledge and Kegan Paul, 1968.

Campbell, K. Body and Mind. New York: Doubleday & Co., Inc., 1970.

Dasgupta, S. A History of Indian Philosophy (Vol. 1). London: Cambridge University Press, 1932.

Duessen, P. The Philosophy of the Upanishads. New York: Dover Publications, Inc., 1966.

Hiriyanna, M. The Essentials of Indian Philosophy. Bombay, India: George Allen & Unwin. (India), 1973.

Prabhavananda, S. Vedic Religion and Philosophy. Madras, India: Sri Rama Krishna Math, 1974.

Taimni, I. K. The Science of Yoga. Adyar, Madras 20, India: Theosophical Publishing House, 1971.

Yogananda, P. Man's Eternal Quest. Los Angeles: Self-Realization Fellowship, 1976.

Yogananda, P. Autobiography of a Yogi. Los Angeles: Self-Realization Fellowship, 1979.

Yukteswar, S. The Holy Science. Los Angeles: Self-Realization Fellowship, 1972.

Solitude, Silence and Personhood

Orlo Strunk, Jr.

Despite the tedious and often pedantic characteristics associated with introductory materials, it seems imperative--given the definitional nature of this conference and its particular topic--that careful attention be paid to perspectives and to what Giorgi (1970) calls approach. If it is indeed our task to take seriously the notion of spirit-centered wholeness, we are surely obligated to be as clear and open as possible relative to the framework and the paradigms from which we struggle to articulate our ideas and our convictions. Nothing can be gained from an Olympian stance or from falling ill to what Sigmund Koch (1981) has so marvelously, and I think accurately, referred to as epistemopathy--a sort of making believe we know when we don't. In fact--as I hope to suggest later on--it may well be that the most difficult and challenging task facing those who would address the issue of spirit-centered wholeness is learning to live creatively with the reality of mystery.

Given, then, the enormity implicit in defining spirit-centered wholeness, the parameters of approach stand in need of at least a skeletal explication.

First, the disciplinary stance I shall take might best be termed that of a contemplative psychology. Although it is true that most of my intellectual life has been spent researching and writing in the area of the psychology of religion, I do not believe that that field of inquiry, given its propensities and current status, provides a particularly rewarding or even an especially friendly atmosphere for the sort of probe I wish to make--although there are recent signs that its project may be undergoing some promising revisioning.[2] This judgment on my part in no sense questions that discipline's potential contributions to a better understanding of such a topic as spirit-centered wholeness or to the possible place of solitude and silence in that understanding. What I am suggesting is that at this time in my life the notion of a contemplative psychology appears to hold richer and more promising contributions than does a psychology of religion.

Although contemplative psychology itself stands constantly in need of formulation and reformulation, for the purpose of this paper Gerald G. May's recent definition of the approach seems especially promising:

> A contemplative psychology is an approach to human experience that maintains that wisdom depends upon a full cooperation of all ways of knowing: observation, logical inference, behavioral learning, and intuition, and it seeks to expand the innate human capacity for intuitive perception. The goal of a contemplative psychology is not the separate autonomy of the individual but the realization of one's essential rootedness in God and relatedness in creation. Its means are not willful mastery but willing surrender. Its resources lie in the comparison of modern psychological understandings with the insights of ancient spiritual traditions of both East and West. And its laboratory is the stillness of the human mind in silence (May, 1982, pp. 26-27).[3]

Secondly, the primary focus for exploring solitude and silence will be that of personhood. Again, this is a conscious preference--one chosen out of a variety of other possibilities, and one, of course, severely questionable from the positions of other foci. Indeed, in our times of cross-cultural awareness and pleas for greater systemic thinking it is quite easy to straddle critically the notion of personhood with the old individualistic censure--the claim that a stress on personhood is ipso facto to fall before a massive and significant scotoma; namely, the failure to realize the paramount and even fateful power of culture and its intricacies. But this, I would argue, is to superficialize and to caricature a potentially rich notion, one which has in fact at various times in intellectual and political history challenged the most ingenious minds. For no matter how systematic we may struggle to be in our thinking, every searcher, sooner or later, is pressed to focus, to admit that her or his conceptual centrosome is this or that. There can be no argument that such foci vary greatly both in intellectual history and in personal predilections. In fact, it is even reasonable to explain our variety of disciplines and respective fields of inquiry as partly at least preoccupations with explications stemming from particular foci.

In this look at solitude and silence as related to the definitional task confronting the larger project of spirit-centered wholeness, I am then suggesting that personhood, and the center of personhood, represents a crucial focus.

In this regard, the recent work of M. Brewster Smith is heuristically helpful; and I shall be noting it in the attempt to explain why it is that the richness of both solitude and silence can be productively grasped in the context of personhood.

Thirdly, and finally, it needs to be noted that besides the backdrop formed by contemporary psychological studies, and particularly by a contemplative psychology, both Western and Eastern religions and the spiritualities often associated with them are implicit in much of my treatment. At the same time, it will be clear in the following exposition that a Western mentality bestrides an Eastern one. This is said neither apologetically nor boastingly--merely descriptively; and, given my own biography, I think, inevitably.

These, then, constitute the parameters of approach --the formal discipline of contemplative psychology in which personhood assumes a focal point with Western and Eastern spiritualities forming the horizon. From this framework an attempt will be made to consider the conditions of solitude and silence, the place they hold in coming to appreciate the natural depth of personhood, the contributions such an understanding might make in defining spirit-centered wholeness, and the potential avenues they hold for further development of the wider project of meaning-searching and the building of a viable praxis.

Personhood

As we all know, personhood has a long and noble place in the history of ideas, particularly in the development of Western philosophy. Equally evidenced is the fact that as a concept, it has suffered mightily in the past several decades. The demise of the person, for example, under the onslaught of the behavioral and social sciences has been well documented (Evans, 1977), and there is little doubt that with some of the most significant conceptualizations of such thinkers as Freud and Marx personalistic categories have been minimal.

It is of course true that much of this demise can be seen not so much as a profound critique of authentic personhood but rather as an attack on an often superficial and even naive presentation of that notion. In some instances, the assault actually has been launched against such terms as "the person" or "the self" or "the soul," all of which imply a thing-ness nowhere near the intricate and depthful dynamism so necessary if the term is to reflect the realities already discovered by poets, philosophers, theologians, mystics, and, more recently, by those who envision psychology as a human science.

In this attempt to explore the nature of a spirit-centered wholeness, I trust this propensity for over-simplification can be avoided, even though it cannot be completely eliminated in any exploration which considers personhood from a limiting stance--although contemplative psychology, I think, does reduce the tendency somewhat. Nor for the particular purpose of this paper is it necessary to explore the many philosophical nuances implicit in any serious consideration of the nature of personhood--a project which still needs doing again in concordance with the contemporary interest of a growing number of psychologists desirous of revisiting person and personhood.[4]

In fact, the personalistic view I am suggesting is partly contained not so much in the context of the technical notion of personhood at all; but rather by the label "selfhood" as it is often used by the psychologist, H. Brewster Smith. In his Presidential Address delivered at the meeting of the American Psychological Association in Toronto in 1978, he characterized selfhood as a label for the criterial features of the human condition which since people have become self-consciously aware of their special place in the world has been a prime puzzle--along with the cosmological puzzle--to which myth, religion, and philosophy always have been concerned. In more detail, Smith (1978, pp. 1053-1054) wrote:

> I am talking . . . about universal features of being a person, distinctive features that we find fascinating and, when we take them seriously, as mysterious as the frontiers of cosmology . . . Selfhood involves being <u>self-aware</u> or <u>reflective</u>; <u>being</u> or <u>having</u> a body; . . . somehow taking into account the <u>boundaries of selfhood</u> at birth and death and feeling a <u>continuity of identity</u> in between; placing oneself in a <u>generational sequence and network of other connected selves</u> while experiencing an <u>irreducible separateness of experience and identity</u>; engaging in joint and individual <u>enterprises</u> in the world with some degree of <u>forethought and afterthought</u> (not just "behaving"); <u>guiding</u> what one does and <u>appraising</u> what one has done at least partly through <u>reflection</u> on one's performance; feeling <u>responsible</u> at least sometimes, for one's actions and holding others responsible for theirs.

It is Smith's contention that such concerns--and others as well--ought to be integral to a truly human psychology; and that there are appropriate perspectives --phylogenetic, cross-cultural, transhistorical, and ontogenetic--which are legitimate avenues for the psychologist to follow.

It is this sort of swirling conceptual caldron that frames a contemplative psychology as well. But it asks further and with some eagerness: In what ways do we come to experience these universal features? How do we as persons discover the sources of such varied and distinctive criterial characteristics? And what difference does it make if indeed a person commits herself or himself to such a view of person?

One suggestion is that we take very seriously the notion that at the center of personhood is a point, a quiet eye, a true Self, where all systems meet and we are laid plain. There is in you and in me a quiet place that truly identifies you as you and me as me. It is what the late Thomas Merton (1968) meant when he spoke of "the heart" as "the deepest psychological ground of one's personality, the inner sanctuary where self-awareness goes beyond analytical reflection." Not only that, but this centerpoint is secret (Strunk, 1976); perhaps even unknowable. As Winnicott (1965, p. 187) has noted:

> In health there is a core of the personality that corresponds to the true self. I suggest that this core never communicates with the world of perceived objects and that the individual person knows that it must never be communicated with or be influenced by external reality. Although healthy persons communicate and enjoy communicating, the other fact is equally true, that each individual is an isolate, permanently noncommunicating, permanently unknown, in fact, unfound.

Thomas Merton's metaphor of the heart, I think, is particularly appropriate in sensing the mystery involved at this level of search.[5] He writes, "Finding our heart and recovering this awareness of our inmost identity implies the recognition that our external, everyday self is to a great extent a mask and a fabrication. It is not our true self. And indeed our true self is not easy to find. It is hidden in obscurity and nothingness at the center where we are in direct dependence on God." (Merton, 1968, p. 20)

What perhaps is even more fascinating in regard to this sort of understanding of the center of personhood is the promise as well as the surprises that it has led not a few searchers to a view in concordance with certain modern cosmological puzzles. In his criticisms of relativity theory, David Bohm, a theoretical physicist, has proposed the notion of an interconnected universe, a kind of holographic relationship in which reality is "undivided wholeness in flowing movement" and where, for instance, mind and matter are not separate substances at all but "different aspects of one whole and unbroken movement." (Bohm, 1980).

A poetic translation of this realization may go something like this:

The sparrow on the stone wall
is the tip of your finger;
and the crow watching from the oak
is the retina of your eye.

Those dark limbs in the morning haze
are the bones that hold your flesh firm;
and the unending grayness above
is the mystery of your soul.

Those two red squirrels scurrying
is the blood rushing through your heart;
you feel their breath against your cheek
and when you move they move with you.

It is not, of course, necessary that the poet's sense, or that of the mystic's, correspond to that of the scientist. Rather what is often surprising and fascinating is that they frequently do.

What, then, are conditions in which such sensitivities are given? What conditions seem to be necessary for one to move toward the heart? And what might we discover there that will assist us in coming to a meaning of at least the beginnings of a definition of spirit-centered wholeness?

Solitude and Silence

Although I will be arguing that solitude and silence are conditions which have inestimable value for such a meaning-searching project, they are but selected examples. There are, of course, a variety of conditions which one could point to as contextual necessities for arriving at a sense of what has been called the givens of existence. But I have chosen solitude and silence for three reasons: First, both conditions hold central places in the history of spirituality, Western and Eastern; secondly, much in contemporary culture not only runs counter to the cultivations of these modes of being but tends to outlaw them completely (Leech, 1977, p. 180); and, thirdly, I have found them to be especially rewarding in my own spiritual quest (Strunk, 1982).

In another place in exploring the notion of privacy, I tried to suggest the contributions potentially available through the condition of being-apart-from-others (Strunk, 1982). I suggested that this condition, often shunned and criticized by a collectivistic mentality, makes a unique contribution of soul-searching and that, when properly understood and lived, is capable of assisting the person in an identification process which adds personal and social dimensions quite beyond those ordinarily discovered in psychological and interpersonal explorations. In one sense that essay was focused essentially on methodological and prescriptive concerns. And although such concerns are not irrelevant to our definitional task, I would like in the space allotted to note two particular discoveries which seem to me to be foundational to any spirit-centered project.

Before turning to these topics, however, I would like to correct an impression which somehow gets expressed whenever privacy or solitude gain a place for discussion. Frequently it is assumed that such a condition is a respite project--a sort of leisurely retreat where one is able to withdraw from the hubbub of daily activities. Although such does indeed constitute one small part of the meaning of solitude, it is unfortunately much too one-sided a view to form the substantial foundation necessary to account for the significant place it has held in the history of spirituality. Rather than argue this point through extensive references to the nature of the solitary life in, for example, the Middle Ages or to the rich and varied expositions of it by ancient desert Fathers, let me quote just a few lines from a contemporary poem written by the New England poet May Sarton (1978, p. 83) which captures well my excursion:

I can tell you that solitude
Is not all exaltation, inner space
Where the soul breathes and work can be done.
Solitude exposes the nerve,
Raises up ghosts.
The past, never at rest, flows through it.

This is not simply a parenthetical notation but a sound discovery which must be counted as part of the solitary condition. I fear we have become so enamored over collectivistic and togetherness values that we stand in real danger of denying the potentialities hidden in the solitary state. As Matthew Kelty (1979, p. 36) so forcefully has put it: "Togetherness does not breed love. It tends rather to strengthen the notion that the problem is other people. Time to be alone guarantees commerce with God and one's heart."

But back to the claim that there are already findings available to us which have come forth from a variety of explorations in personhood and which need to be included in any comprehensive attempt to define, if only heuristically, spirit-centered wholeness.

The first such discovery is that at the center of personhood is an aura of willingness, not willfulness. Although there are subtle differences here to be dealt with, they are crucial and telling. In exploring these differences, Gerald May (1982, p. 6) has aptly put it this way:

> . . . willingness implies a surrendering of one's self-separateness, an entering-into, an immersion in the deepest processes of life itself. It is a realization that one already is a part of some ultimate cosmic process and it is a commitment to participation in that process. In contrast, willfulness is the setting of oneself apart from the fundamental essence of life in an attempt to master, direct, control, or otherwise manipulate existence. More simply, willingness is saying yes to the mystery of being alive in each moment. Willfulness is saying no, or perhaps more commonly, "Yes, but . . ."

Given our propensities for willfulness, this discovery holds great significance in the formation of a wholistic stance, no matter our professional interests or our pockets of praxis. Partly the realization may be explicated within the notion of a particular sort of surrender, or, perhaps more accurately, by a depthful understanding of the complementarity of mastery and surrender (Fisher, 1983).

Although it is certainly true that solitude and silence provide an often demonstrated condition for such a discovery, it is also true, I believe, that the trough of surrender--or of willingness as over against willfulness--is itself discovery and constitutes a necessary dimension of any authentic spirit-centered notion.

The same may be said of the condition of silence. Again, we are confronted with a massive literature, both Western and Eastern, which calls us to take more seriously the place of silence in the realization of our spiritual center. A minuscule but typical sample within a particular spiritual tradition may be seen in this brief excerpt from one of Jacob Boehme's (1978, p. 171) tracts:

1. The student said to the master: "How may I come to the supersensual life so that I can see God and hear Him speak?" The master said: "If you can sweep up for a moment into that in which no creature dwells, you can hear what God speaks."
2. The student said: "Is that near or far?" The master said: "It is in you. If you could be silent from all willing and thinking for one hour you would hear God's inexpressible words."

3. The student said: "How can I hear when I remain silent in thinking and willing?" The master said: "When you remain silent from the thinking and willing of self, the eternal hearing, seeing and speaking will be revealed in you, and God will see and hear through you. Your own hearing, willing and seeing hinders you so that you do not see and hear God."
4. The student said: "With what shall I see and hear God, since He is above nature and creature?" The master said: "When you move silently then you are that which God was before nature and creature, (that) out of which He created your nature and creature. Then you will hear and see with that which God saw and heard in you before your own willing, seeing and hearing began."

In a more modern vein and from the perspective of a contemplative psychology--and keeping in mind our contemporary inclination for willful noise-making -- silence is perhaps the most dramatic avenue for discovering the mystery at the heart of personhood and beyond. In Gaston Backelard's (1964, pp. 43-44) beautiful phenomenology of the house, he turns at one point to Henri Basco quoting as follows:

> There is nothing like silence to suggest a sense of unlimited space. Sounds lend color to space and confer a sort of sound body upon it. But absence of sound leaves it quite purc and, in the silence, we are seized with the sensation of something vast and deep and boundless . . .

We are reminded here of the many ways in which silence and solitude helped to reinforce what some would count as the heart of Christianity--that is, the mystery of the paradox of divine revelation (Hardy, 1976). In the Sanjuanist tradition, for example, the notion of the hidden God takes on a power quite beyond our ordinary conceptualizations. In commenting of Fran Juan's famous poem, La Noche Oscura, the eminent scholar, Richard P. Hardy, Professor of Spirituality at Saint Paul University in Ottawa, has noted that "only solitude and silence in the perspective of Fran Juan can enable man to the positive extending of his open hands to be grasped and thus led by God to fulfillment" (Hardy, 1976, p. 252).

At the very heart of this approach lies, of course, the mystery element of God. "It is," continues Professor Hardy, "the hidden God who loves and cares for man. It is the hidden God who brings him to Himself. It is the hidden God who is searched for by man. Because of this quality, man, who is given to see Him, comes to enter a whole life devoted to seeking out the God who hides" (Hardy, 1976, pp. 261-262). And in another place:

> Silence in the Christian perspective is seen as the reality which is meant to open oneself to the God who comes. In silence one can be attentive to all that is present. The child knows that in playing "hide and seek," for example, silence is of the utmost importance. And this is so because he knows that sounds draw the attention of a person to its source. Thus, the child would be discovered immediately if he made a noise. Despite the banality of the example chosen here,it does reflect the fact that when man hears sound he is versed in the origin of that sound and consequently he is drawn away from the intense

listening stature for which silence allows . . . (Hardy, 1976, p. 221).

This is, of course, a perspective grounded in the recognition of the reality of mystery. And to our modern ears--conditioned powerfully by a religion, a science, and a technology often prone to image a god who controls all but who is controlled by us--it is not an especially popular viewpoint. And this is, of course, one of the reasons we often do indeed avoid both conditions of silence and solitude, sensing--if only vaguely--that they hold auras of surrender and especially of mystery.

Yet, if spirit-centered wholeness is to be sensed in an authentic way, these particular learnings must be taken into account in the definitional task.

Summary and Overview

Before turning to a few of the avenues of search which such a perspective may imply, let me summarize my thesis to this point: In our attempts to come to a heuristic definition of spirit-centered wholeness, I have suggested that a promising notion is that of personhood where we discover those universal and distinctive realities which make us truly human; and that the conditions of solitude and silence hold a special place in this discovery process. Not only do such conditions hold methodological aids--as has been dramatically demonstrated again and again in both Western and Eastern spiritualities--they have pointed consistently to the surfacing of at least two discoveries: (1) the necessity of surrender as a complementary force to the common stance of mastery or willfulness, and (2) the reality of a mystery which must chaperon all our discoveries and understandings. I have implied that although such a project of inquiry may take place within a variety of disciplinary contexts, the perspective of a contemplative psychology offers an especially promising one.

As to avenues of research and investigation which seem to me to flow easily from this sort of picture, I note at least five which are particularly evident and which hold special interest to me:

1. We are required as never before in intellectual history to take seriously the paradigmatic foundations of our various projects of inquiry and our schema of praxis. No longer, for instance, is it possible or responsible for such important areas as psychology and psychiatry to avoid dealing with their assumptional systems and their philosophical and/or theological foundations and fictions. The implications of this acknowledgment are many; but certainly one is the necessity for greater interdisciplinary dialogue and mutual critiquing across disciplines.

2. We are required to deal with the exceedingly perplexing question of what difference it makes <u>what</u> perspective we hold relative to praxis. If, for instance, a helper--no matter his or her professional area--has assimilated an enlightened notion of spirit-centered wholeness--what precisely and generally are the practical consequences of such a stance? Admittedly an age-old problem of the relationship between personhood and behavior, it nevertheless remains a crucial area of exploration.

3. Despite the massive literature dealing with solitude and silence--much of it framed within religious systems--we desperately need new phenomenologies of the experience of solitude and the experience of

silence as they are embedded in a technological age which is evolving new and different levels of consciousness in nearly every area of life, from religious experiences, feminist expressions, minority claims, political urgings, etc.

4. We must examine with greater care and honesty the authenticity of praxis claims in all those projects which promise greater health or cure or growth or individuation or self-actualization or healing or salvation. Partly this means facing up to the nature and limits of the knowledge generated by our sundry theories and practices.

In this regard, several specific areas especially stand in need of critical assessment, I believe: modern psychotherapy, contemporary movements in pastoral counseling, and spiritual direction and guidance.

Already some sober warnings have been made relative to the totalization propensity of much of contemporary psychotherapy (e.g., Kovel, 1976, pp. 254-255). The field stands in need of critical and enlightened assessment as to whether it is indeed conceptually and operationally capable of dealing with the sort of issues implicit in a notion of spirit-centered wholeness.

Pastoral counseling, as well as pastoral psychotherapy, stands in need of a similar scrutiny. Its visioning has faltered and has, I believe, slipped into a psychosocial mentality which falls considerably short of the sort of paradigm implicit in a spirit-centered project (Strunk, 1982).

Spiritual direction and guidance with its long and established traditions seems to have survived its near demise of two decades ago and is now interfacing with certain contemporary psychotherapies and with some expressions of pastoral counseling (e.g., Culligan, 1980, 1983; Barry and Connolly, 1982). In terms of the topic of this definitional conference, it appears to hold real promise; but its often close ties to specific traditional religious systems--a factor often counted by many as an essential ingredient--needs to be researched with greater vigor as secular modes of spirituality become more and more prevalent in our times.

5. It seems to me that the two great puzzles of both Western and Eastern religions and spiritualities--the human soul and the cosmos--need to be addressed in concordance. With the theoretical advances in contemporary physics, for example, and with the growing openness of certain movements in contemporary psychology, possibilities for soul/cosmos correlations appear breathtaking and exciting.

Needless to say, such avenues have dozens of sub-issues and problems, both theoretical and practical. We are, I think, being called to enter what Bachelard (1969) has called the "domain of the superlative" where we are at times required to leave the positive for the imaginary, to listen to the poets as well as to the scientist.

Footnotes

1. I wish to thank Dr. John L. Maes, Executive Director of The Danielsen Institute, Boston University, for his support in the preparation of this paper. I am particularly appreciative of his willingness to provide me with travel funds for attending this Conference. I am as well appreciative of those colleagues and graduate students at Boston University who offered comments and suggestions on an earlier draft of this paper.
2. It is encouraging to note that in 1983 at least three texts in the psychology of religion have been planned for publication by three major publishers. Perhaps of even greater significance is the growing number of doctoral dissertations being written in this field by young scholars. Presently, for example, I am serving as a First Reader on one (Stewart, 1983) which seems to me to be a depthful and exciting response to the field from a Jungian perspective.
3. Of course, there are many other scholars developing a variety of forms of contemplative psychology, perhaps not always using the designation. Certainly the many works of Morton Kelsey, for instance--familiar to those involved in the development of the Institute for Religion and Wholeness--would be an eminent example within a Christian stream of spirituality.
4. Having been weaned on Boston personalism in both my undergraduate and graduate education, I am especially sensitive to the intellectual power of the notion of person as it has been explicated by an armada of thinkers at the turn of the century. It is therefore encouraging to note signs of resurrection of personalism as a philosophic stance. My hope would be that as mainstream psychology moves closer to a willingness to explore more depthfully its roots and assumptional fictions, it will discover in this particular philosophic stream some useful ideas.
5. Apparently this same metaphor holds similar power in certain Oriental cultures as well. Benjamin Pao, a Ph.D. candidate at Boston University, is presently writing a dissertation on the Chinese concept of heart (hsis) and already has uncovered a rich array of meanings related to that term.

References

Bachelard, G. The Poetics of Space. Boston: Beacon Press, 1964.

Barry, W. A., & Connolly, W. J. The Practice of Spiritual Direction. New York: The Seabury Press. 1982.

Boehme, J. Jacob Boehme: The Way of Christ. New York: Paulist Press, 1978.

Bohm, D. Wholeness and the Implicate Order. London: Routledge & Kegan Paul, 1980.

Culligan, K. G. (Ed.) Spiritual Direction: Contemporary Readings. Locust Valley, New York: Living Flame Press, 1983.

Culligan, K. G. Toward a Contemporary Model of Spiritual Direction: A Comparative Study of Saint John of the Cross and Carl R. Rogers. Ephemerides Carmeliticae, 1980, 31, 29-90.

Evans, C. S. Preserving the Person: A Look at the Human Sciences. Downers Grove, Ill: InterVarsity Press, 1977.

Fisher, S. C. Surrender in Pastoral Psychotherapy: Towards a Psychological Understanding. Unpublished doctoral dissertation, Boston University, 1983.

Giorgi, A. Psychology as a Human Science: A Phenomenologically based Approach. New York: Harper & Row, 1970.

Hardy, R. P. The Hidden God and Juan de la Cruz. Ephemerides Carmeliticae, 1976, 27, 241-262.

Hardy, R. P. "Silencio Divino": A Sanjuanist Study. Eglise et Theologie (has accents on this), 1976a, 7, 219-233.

Kelty, M. Flute Solo. Kansas City, MO: Andrews & McNeely, 1979.

Koch, S. The Nature and Limits of Psychological Knowledge. American Psychologist, 1981, 36, 257-269.

Kovel, J. A Complete Guide to Therapy: From Psychoanalysis to Behavior Modification. New York: Pantheon Books, 1976.

Leech, K. Soul Friend: The Practice of Christian Spirituality. San Francisco, Calif.: Harper & Row, 1977.

May, G. G. Will and Spirit: A Contemplative Psychology. New York: Harper & Row, 1982.

Merton, T. Contemplative Prayer. Garden City, N.J.: Image Books, Doubleday & Co., 1968.

Sarton, May. Selected Poems of May Sarton. New York: W. W. Norton, 1978.

Smith, M. B. Perspectives on Selfhood. American Psychologist, 1978, 33, 1053-1059.

Stewart, R. D. Archetypal Hermeneutics: The Psychology of Religion and the Religion of Psychology. Unpublished doctoral dissertation, Boston University, 1983. In preparation.

Strunk, O., Jr. The Secret Self. Nashville, Tenn.: Abingdon Press, 1976.

Strunk, O., Jr. Privacy: Experience, Understanding, Expression. Washington, D.C.: The University Press of America, 1982.

Strunk, O., Jr. The Role of Visioning in the Pastoral Counseling Movement. Pastoral Psychology, 1982, 31, 7-18.

Winnicott, D. M. Communicating and Not Communicating: Leading to a Study of Certain Opposites. In The Maturation Processes and the Facilitating Environment. New York: International Universities Press, 1965.

INSTITUTIONAL WHOLENESS

Religious Community and Human Wholeness: Perspectives from the Sociology of Religion

Donald E. Miller

To address the subject of human wholeness from a sociological perspective involves one, almost inevitably, in accenting the social nature of humankind. In the pages that follow, my bias will be evident that I see human wholeness as integrally related both to the individual's experience of community as well as the moral health of the larger society. I will also argue that the religious community has considerable potential as a setting in which human wholeness can be cultivated (cf. Miller, 1981). It will be evident that I do not speak for all sociologists of religion. This would be impossible since the field is nearly as diverse as society itself. Nevertheless, I will attempt to delineate some common themes that are developed by a number of sociologists and also note some of the methodological issues at stake in understanding the relationship between religion and human wholeness.

In the first section of the paper I will examine several functionalist definitions of religion and show how a possible bridge can be made between religion and human wholeness. In the second section, I will briefly survey some of the major classical theorists who have commented on the relationship between religion and the individual and/or society. The third section of the paper will note the thought of several contemporary writers and their views of religion's role in modern society. Finally, I will offer some evaluative remarks and a few personal reflections on the interconnection between religion and wholeness.

Defining Religion

A number of sociologists define religion in terms of its functions. Robert Bellah (1970:21), for example, states that religion is "a set of symbolic forms and acts that relate man to the ultimate conditions of his existence." Similarly, J. Milton Yinger (1970:7) states that "religion . . . can be defined as a system of beliefs and practices by means of which a group of people struggles with (the) ultimate problems of human life." Implicit in these two definitions is the idea that the problem of meaning is central to the daily struggle with death, suffering, and the purpose for living.

Since we are born into a world with pre-existing systems of meaning, many people seek answers to these problems of life within the context of an institutionalized meaning system. Indeed, in Yinger's view, religious beliefs and rituals are created and crafted by those who have felt the problems of life most intensely. But for a variety of reasons, not everyone finds satisfactory answers at the local Baptist, Catholic, or Presbyterian church. So some people innovate, putting together their own collage of meaning systems. Others find their identity in a "secular religion," such as psychoanalysis or Marxism. From a functionalist perspective, however, the question is not so much <u>whether</u> an individual is religious, but <u>how</u> are they religious. The presumption is that every individual needs a reason to live as well as legitimation for the values they espouse.

From a functional perspective, religion and human wholeness are integrally related; wholeness requires interaction with, or commitment to, a set of norms and beliefs (sustained in ritual or performative expression). The only person who is not religious is one who is not involved in reflecting on his or her purpose for living. In short, my assumption is that one cannot be "whole" unless one allows questions of meaning and purpose to be at the very center of one's everyday experience. Such a concern does not guarantee wholeness, but it is, I believe, a prerequisite to wholeness.

Wholeness involves integration of the personality around a central myth or belief system. A "life myth" enables one to live and work with a sense of purpose and order. Because life myths tend to be grounded by individuals in appeals to what is "really real," "truly true," or "the way things were meant to be," God-language is often a part of the official justification of one's values. In contemporary times, however, one's vision of life's purpose and order may just as likely be rooted in ecological principles, or biological, psychological, or political goals. To the extent that these principles or goals take on an absolutistic quality, I believe they are the functional equivalent of traditional religious legitimations.

Classical Figures

In this next section we will examine several major theorists dealing with the role and function of religion. Their views will range from stating that religion is entirely a social by-product, to saying that religion is detrimental to the human spirit, to arguing historically that the effects of religion must be examined on a case by case basis. In this survey, we will note each theorist's view of the modern world in our assessment of their contribution to a theory of human wholeness.

Emile Durkheim

For Emile Durkheim (1858-1917), religion had quite a different role in primitive societies than it does in modern society. In primitive societies there was very little personal individuality, says Durkheim (1964:92). Members of the group held the same values, the same things were held sacred, and social cohesion was based on congruence of attitude and beliefs. The object of worship, said Durkheim, was society: the collectively held beliefs which allow for group social cohesion (what Durkheim (1964:79) called the "collective conscience"). God, thought Durkheim, was society transfigured into a religious symbol. Religious ritual was a major contributor to the experience of social solidarity.

> In the midst of an assembly animated by a common passion, we become susceptible of acts and sentiments of which we are incapable when reduced to our own forces; and when the assembly is dissolved and when, finding ourselves alone again, we fall back to our ordinary level, we are then able to measure the height to which we have been raised above ourselves (1965:240).

This experience of "creative effervescence" is what members of the group identify as "the sacred." Such ritual moments are significant, for " . . . the coming together of a number of men associated in the same life results in disengaging new energies, which transform each of them" (1965:252).

Using primitive society as a paradigm, Durkheim believed that although religion's role had greatly dissipated in modern society, nevertheless societies continue to maintain themselves, at least in part, through group celebration (interdependence, because of the high division of labor, being the other source of social solidarity).

> There can be no society which does not feel the need of upholding and reaffirming at regular intervals the collective sentiments and the collective ideas which make its unity and its personality (1965:475).

It is from this key Durkheimian notion that Robert Bellah (1967) built his now famous civil religion concept. Will Herberg (1960), some years before Bellah, argued that "the American Way of Life" was at the core of religious celebration in the United States.

The important idea to be drawn from Durkheim for our purposes is that society cannot exist without its individual members sharing certain core values. Likewise, the individual cannot exist today without society. Human wholeness is to be defined in terms of the individual being integrated into society, performing their appropriate function and thereby contributing to the maintenance of society. In spite of Durkheim's conviction that modern societies are bound together more by mutual interdependence than likeness of values, Durkheim never lost sight of the fact that the individual owes his or her very existence to society: "the individual is not sufficient unto himself, it is from society that he receives everything necessary to him" (1964:228).

Generalizing from Durkheim about the relationship between religion and human wholeness, it is fair to say that the individual and society are deeply intertwined. In primitive society, this connection was celebrated in religious ritual; in rite and ceremony the individual lost his/her individuality and merged with the group experiencing "the sacred" in the process (the "sacred" being the collective sentiments in which group solidarity is rooted). In modern society, the risk of anomie and alienation is greatly heightened. In Durkheim's (1964:172) words, there has emerged "a cult in behalf of personal dignity." Modern society is characterized by a highly evolved division of labor. Nevertheless, a vague but clearly definable "civil religion" remains. At some level, all group members share some common values, but "little by little, political, economic, scientific functions free themselves from the religious function, constitute themselves apart and take on a more and more acknowledged temporal character" (1964:169).

> As all the other beliefs and all the other practices take on a character less and less religious, the individual becomes the object of a sort of religion (1964:172).

Such a statement, however, must be placed next to Durkheim's (1964:405) statement: "The only power which can serve to moderate individual egotism is the power of the group." In short, the individual, religion (albeit civil religion), and society all exist in a potentially complementary relationship. Human wholeness depends on maintaining a proper balance: individuality has its place, but within a community that is bound together through interdependence as well as the social cement of rite and ritual.

Marx and Freud

Even though Durkheim held a rather reductionistic view regarding the "spirit" that enervates religion and society, he nevertheless saw the importance of religion and did not dismiss it as a mere hallucination. Marx (Marx & Engels, 1964) and Freud (1961a, 1961b), in contrast, thought that the time had come to do away with religion. In terms of human wholeness, they both believed that religion enslaves individuals--either by allegiance to an irrational authority (Freud) or in dependence as an opiate (Marx). In neither case was religion contributing to the maturity or growth of either the individual or society.

Freud, to repeat the widely known formulation, believed that God was a projection which functions in the midst of the pervasive human feelings of fear, insecurity and anxiety. Marx, likewise, saw religion as a source of consolation, offering to the poor and disinherited a promise of a better life to come. Marx did not deny the distress of the oppressed, but he concurred with Feuerback that God is the projection of one's own qualities and powers; theology is a mystified form of anthropology.

So with Marx and Freud we see two major figures who believed that religion diminishes the human spirit, that it enslaves them to irrational authority, and drains them of their own sense of virtue and control. Religion offers security and control, but it is a false security: it is time to mature, grow up, cast off the yoke that perpetuates impoverishment. The primary difference separating Freud and Marx is that Freud had few illusions about human potential. Freud was a realist. He did not believe in the possibility of a salvation external to the self. Psychoanalysis does not promise happiness, only more freedom of choice and self-determination. If human wholeness was to be achieved, it was in the art of self-creation, casting off external restrictions, living a life unfettered by guilt, inhibitions, and unconscious motivations. Marx, on the other hand, was a utopian. He quested for a perfect classless society where no alienation would exist, where all people would be equal; where the coercive apparatus of police, courts, and army would be unnecessary. Human wholeness would be a direct function of social conditions and so he struggled by prophesy and class analysis to bring in the new society.

At one level, it is possible to affirm the view of Marx and Freud. _If_ religion enslaves, is authoritarian, and saps people of the motive for achieving a just society, then religion should be abolished. On the other hand, however, one must ask whether Marx or Freud were seeing religion in its full range of expression and complexity. Freud's most direct reports of religion were from neurotic patients who one can imagine employed religion in a very dependent manner. Marx also took too narrow a view of religion in not recognizing its potential for change. He would be surprised, I suspect, to see Liberation Theologians employing his class analysis. The contribution of Marx and Freud to our discussion of human wholeness is in helping us to be discriminating in talking about religion. Not all religious forms are the same: some religious expressions are more conducive to closedness than openness, authoritarianism than reasonableness, repression than freedom. On the other hand, it is difficult to forget the example of a Martin Luther King, a Gandhi, or a host of others for whom religion was an empowering force, not a source of quietism. Even some of those who are mystically minded, such as Thomas Merton, have gone a long way toward uniting an inner and outer life, the life of action and the life of reflection.

Max Weber

It is difficult to ignore Max Weber in any discussion of the sociology of religion, but at the same time it is equally difficult to give a neat summary of a few central thoughts on his view of religion. Weber was a historian who reveled in details. Personally he identified himself as "religiously unmusical," and yet he spent the better part of his life studying religion and documenting its impact. He disagreed with Marx that religion was merely a reflection of the economic order. Surely religion and economics always interact, but religion, in his view, may provide the ideas that structure the economic order. Weber's famed Protestant ethic thesis is a single case study examining the impact of religion on the social order. _The Protestant Ethic and the Spirit of Capitalism_ (1958) should be read, however, alongside of his studies of the religions of China, India, and Judaism. In the former case study, religion had a decidedly modernizing impact; in the latter cases, religion had a more traditional orientation and impact.

One formulation by Weber (1946:323-359) that directly impacts on the subject of human wholeness is his four-fold typology of salvation. Weber, a master of typological analysis, saw four patterns: (1) innerworldly asceticism, (2) otherworldly asceticism, (3) innerworldly mysticism, and (4) otherworldly mysticism. It is the category of innerworldly asceticism that he identified with the Protestant work ethic. The innerworldly ascetic is one who transfers the seriousness of discipline and work in the monastery to work in the world. The Protestant ethic thesis is too widely known to bear repeating in this context, except to remind the reader that Benjamin Franklin is Weber's secular exemplar of the innerworldly ascetic, especially his views on time and money.

Without elaborating Weber's typology, it is important to note Weber's pessimism about the modern world, for it is this aspect of his thought that bears most directly on the subject of human wholeness. At the end of The Protestant Ethic, Weber (1958:181-82) comments:

> For when asceticism was carried out of monastic cells into everyday life, and began to dominate worldly morality, it did its part in building the tremendous cosmos of the modern economic order. This order is now bound to the technical and economic conditions of machine production which today determine the lives of all the individuals who are born into this mechanism, not only those directly concerned with economic acquisition, with irresistible force. Perhaps it will so determine them until the last ton of fossilized coal is burnt. In Baxter's view the care for external goods should only lie on the shoulders of the "saint like a light cloak, which can be thrown aside at any moment." But fate decreed that the cloak should become an iron cage.

> Since asceticism undertook to remodel the world and to work out its ideals in the world, material goods have gained an increasing and finally an inexorable power over the lives of men as at no previous period in history.
>
> No one knows who will live in this cage in the future, or whether at the end of this tremendous development entirely new prophets will arise, or there will be a great rebirth of old ideas and ideals, or, if neither, mechanized petrification, embellished with a sort of convulsive self-importance. For of the last stage of this cultural development, it might well be truly said, "Specialists without spirit, sensualists without fear; this nullity imagines that it has attained a level of civilization never before achieved.

Weber was a pessimist. Far from the functionalist/consensualist model of Durkheim, Weber saw society as dominated by conflict with different interest groups each attempting to gain advantage over the other. But it wasn't just the classic duel of one group against the other that disturbed Weber (1946:196-264), it was that there is a mounting pattern of "disenchantment," of rationalization, of routinization, of bureaucratization that characterizes every aspect of life from business to religion. There is an emerging cult of efficiency in which the world which has been created is a dreary, flat, utilitarian realm that strips people of their very soul. Religion is being replaced by science, the trained expert for the cultivated person of letters; machines are ousting the skilled handworker, traditional judicial wisdom is being replaced by a mountain of legal codes. Weber

(1946:128) prophesied: "Not summer's bloom lies ahead of us, but rather a polar night of icy darkness and hardness." About the bureaucrat, Weber (1946:228) commented: "In the great majority of cases, he is only a single cog in an ever-moving mechanism which prescribes to him an essentially fixed route of march." Regarding bureaucracy more generally, Weber (1946:215) stated:

> Its specific nature, which is welcomed by capitalism, develops the more perfectly the more the bureaucracy is "dehumanized," the more completely it succeeds in eliminating from official business love, hatred, and all purely personal, irrational, and emotional elements which escape calculation.

Human wholeness in the modern age? Weber was pessimistic. He was particularly sceptical of artificial means of trumping up intimacy.

> The fate of our times is characterized by rationalization and intellectualization and, above all, by the disenchantment of the world. Precisely the ultimate and most sublime values have retreated from public life either into the transcendental realm of mystic life or into the brotherliness of direct and personal relations. It is not accidental that our greatest art is intimate and not monumental, nor is it accidental that today only within the smallest and intimate circles, in personal human situations, in *pianissimo*, something is pulsating that corresponds to the prophetic pneuma, which in former times swept through the great communities like a firebrand, welding them together (1946:155).

In a word, Weber feared the death of genuine community. The role for the charismatic prophet had declined. The historic religions had lost their authority. Somewhat grudgingly he offered his respect to those who could not stand up to the times and returned to the church.

> To the persons who cannot bear the fate of the times like a man, one must say: may he rather return silently, without the usual publicity built-up of renegades, but simply and plainly. The arms of the old churches are opened widely and compassionately for him. After all, they do not make it hard for him (1946:155).

Personally, Weber (1946:156) went in search of "the demon who holds the fibers of his very life," rather than seek refuge in religion. Human wholeness, then, is not an easy task, as is witnessed to by Weber's own mental breakdown at age thirty-three.

In the consideration of human wholeness, Weber importantly introduces the workplace into our discussion. It is not technology which Weber feared, but the impersonality of the management process that accompanies it. Weber also introduces for our discussion the broad concept of the "spirit of the age" and its bearing on everything from our attitude toward work to our relationship to family and religion. Weber's genius is that in the midst of detailed analysis, he could perceive a pattern and identify it through the creation of types and the specification of exemplars of an age. Surely we have much to learn from Weber on a purely methodological basis, irrespective of its prophetic pronouncements.

The Modern Age

One thing that can be said about the classical theorists is that they were wrong on at least one point: religion has not disappeared; indeed, it seems to be pulsating in America at nearly every turn. It would be a mistake, however, to say that nothing has changed, or that their prophesies were totally without merit. Religion may not have disappeared, but its social role has certainly undergone alterations.

Perhaps no one has told the story of the modern age and religion much better than Peter Berger (1969:105-171). In the next few paragraphs I wish to give the flavor of some of the contemporary discussion on modernity by beginning with Berger and then looking very briefly at several other theorists--Robert Bellah, Thomas Luckmann, and Phillip Rieff--and also one contemporary novel.

In The Homeless Mind, Berger (1973) and his co-authors argue that the central fact of the modern individual's existence is the relativization of traditional religious symbol systems. People in the modern world are constantly bombarded with multiple world views. The explosion of the media showers us with images of life from across the globe. To survive, one comes to assume that this is just one more view among many. None are final; none are absolute. Even the person-on-the-street has come to understand that truth claims are conditioned by time and place and more than not reflect the direct self-interest of those who are proclaiming them. Given our mobility of body and mind, we have entered an era of cynicism and relativism. The result is a type of "homelessness" in which all is relative; there is no place to stand with assurance. Everything is in process--developing, changing, moving, being managed--and the result, says Berger, is not an abstract feeling of relativity, but an existential crisis of lostness, nausea, anxiety. Who is the real me? What do I stand for? What can I call true or real?

Robert Bellah (1964) sees, somewhat less pessimistically, a grand pattern of religious evolution which reflects a change from magic and mystery, to authority and system, to an individualized and personalistic view which says that the only truth is what feels right to me. Religion is personal and private. Reason or tradition is no longer authoritative. Bellah (1970:203) quotes the poet Wallace Stevens as expressing the sentiment of the age:

> The final belief is to believe in a fiction, which you know to be a fiction, there being nothing else. The exquisite truth is to know that it is a fiction and that you believe in it willingly.

Bellah thinks religious symbols will continue to play a role in modern society, but they will be used by those who know that they are symbols, not abstract statements of truth--but windows, avenues, conduits to the Truth.

Thomas Luckmann (1967) complements Berger and Bellah in viewing the contemporary individual as a "buyer" who confronts cultural and religious symbol systems, purchasing from them that which fulfills one's private needs. The social world, in his view, offers an incredibly rich assortment of alternative symbols and styles from which the individual may construct his or her own belief system and way of life. Religion, like one's personal identity, becomes a "private affair." Churches and temples are in the heretofore unprecedented position of marketing their wares in a competitive and open arena. The one with the authority in our age is the individual, not the institution or group.

Phillip Rieff (1966) has typified the modern individual in what he calls "Psychological Man." This is a person who is opposed to the constricting communal purposes inherent in tradition or communal life. They have taken themselves, their own self-fulfillment, as the ultimate project. If there is something sacred, it is the "self." These are people, says Rieff, who are much more interested in being "pleased" than being "saved." Book religions are a thing of the past. No prophet is going to denounce these people, stopping their individualistic celebrations of themselves. Character? Truth? Faith? These are words from the old culture. Therapeutic man has put behind him or her the restrictions inherent in such terms.

In concluding this brief look at theorists of the modern age, it is perhaps well to note a novel, The Dice Man, which presents in graphic imagery, if not overdrawn symbolism, the modern character type. Luke Rhinehart, a thirty-two year old psychiatrist, is the central figure in this sophisticated, mildly pornographic book. Bright, successful and bored, he begins to live his life by the caste of a die (singular for dice). To every situation, every significant choice, he writes down six alternatives, some safe, some outrageous, some romantically dangerous. Having identified his choices, he throws the die, following "religiously" the randomized alternative that presents itself. As he lives by the caste of the die his boredom and depression vanish. Life takes on new meaning. It works so well that he introduces "dice therapy" to his patients, many of whom are suffering from his same malady of depression, free-floating anxiety, and boredom. When he is finally reprimanded by the American Psychiatric Association, he offers three defenses for his innovative procedures. Quoting the words of Luke Rhinehart (1971) at his trial:

1. In a multivalent society, the multiple personality is the only one which fulfills. Each of us has a hundred suppressed potential selves which never let us forget that no matter how mightily we step along the single path of our personality, our deepest desire is to be multiple: to play many roles.
2. Our Western psychologies try to solve (people's problems) by urging (them) to suppress (their) natural multiplicity and build a single dominant self to control others.
3. The purpose (of Dice Therapy) is to destroy the personality. We wish to create in its place a multiple personality: an individual inconsistent, unreliable and progressively schizoid.

Berger, Bellah, Luckmann, Rieff, and in near comic form, Luke Rhinehart, provide us with overlapping images of what it means to live in contemporary society. The picture is surely not one of wholeness; rather it is a picture of fragmentation and alienation, of a world in which ultimates have faded into "mere perspectives," and self-centeredness is prized as a virtue. Extracting from the authors just discussed, several basepoints suggest themselves as important to the discussion of human wholeness.

1. We live in a pluralistic world.
2. The relativization of world views is a predictable response to the experience of pluralism.
3. Truth claims are viewed as workable "fictions," helpful, but not ultimately compelling.
4. There is no authority outside of the self;

truth is a matter of feeling, intuition, perspective.

5. Institutional claims to authority are honored so long as they coincide with personal sentiment; guilt is a function of violating self-imposed standards, not societal or ultimate claims.
6. Unity and cohesion of world view are less important than whether something is "interesting" or entertaining.

Surely not everyone fits the above portrait. For example, one may ask about fundamentalists and Moonies, the Moral Majority and the Islamic Revolution--are they not counter examples? Perhaps they are, but it is also possible to see such devotees of absolutism as part of a backlash to the social fragmentation of modern society. Far from escaping the influence of modernity, members of such groups have fled into their communal associations and rigid fundamentalism as a self-protective measure, unable to exist in the wilderness of ambiguity and uncertainty. More characteristic of what is happening in religious communities is the therapeutic character of many "successful" churches and temples which offer forgiveness without penance. Only slightly more expressive of the modern age are those religious groups, many of them "electronic churches," that identify religious commitment with material blessing, upward social mobility, and an undiscriminating Americanism. One might also ask about the 60% of the American population who are not in church on a typical Sunday morning. Have they found salvation in affluence? Or have they given up all hope of living a whole life and instead are sleep-walking in quiet desperation, nearly unaware that there are dreams to be imagined and a more promising life to be pursued.

Evaluation

In concluding, it is perhaps important to indicate some of the limitations of the sociological approach to human wholeness. First, it must be remembered that sociology is a descriptive discipline, not a normative one. Methodologically, most sociologists at least pay lipservice to Max Weber's dictum that social science should be value-free. Thus, although Weber and nearly every sociologist would agree that all investigation and description is done from a specific set of assumptions, the task of the sociologist is much more diagnostic than curative. Narrowly defining their task, sociologists engage in description and analysis rather than evaluation or normative pronouncement. As a matter of fact, however, description and evaluation quite naturally complement each other and the great theorists have almost always moved, at some point, beyond mere description and into normative evaluation, some drawing extensive blueprints for the reformation of society. In these concluding pages, I want to change hats myself and become more normative, even rather personal. But first let me summarize the argument to this point.

We began with the assumption that human wholeness is tied up with the question of meaning and that religion and wholeness are linked together to the extent that religion is viewed as being rooted in the quest for meaning. Next we examined several different theories of the relationship between religion and the individual or society. Then we noted some images of the individual and religion in the modern world. The question presently at hand, I believe, is, "Where do we go from here?"

First, I reject the possibility of returning to some agrarian past where things were less complex. Likewise, I reject establishing an authoritarian religious order or political order that is based on a nostalgic image of a time when perfect harmony prevailed. Going backwards breeds totalitarian rule and is usually more repressive than the conditions it seeks to mitigate. So, in my view, the only alternative is forward. But here I stumble, because I have no blueprint; at best I can confess some of my own directions.

My premise in seeking a way forward is to say that I think pluralism is here to stay and for that reason relativism will continue to plague us. With the explosion in home computer technology, the burgeoning of satellites--the increased ability to store and transmit information--I see the world shrinking and our diversity being more and more apparent at the same time that some of our commonality is more manifest (i.e., we all ache when we are hungry, we all wince when we are shot, we all mourn when our child dies). Perhaps our ability to be closer to each other through the medium of technology will shatter some of the divisiveness of ethnocentrism and elitism. Perhaps barriers between persons will be lowered at the same time that we learn to acknowledge our differences. Relativism, and the awareness of how all meaning systems are socially rooted, might be a blessing in disguise. Tentatively I want to embrace at least some of what technology is doing for us. Perhaps a new tolerance and appreciation of diversity will result. This is the optimistic vision of the new technology.

What happens, however, to the question of "homelessness" in the great wilderness of an urban, technologically sophisticated society? What about the anxiety, emptiness, and meaninglessness that Berger and others have noted? A partial answer, I believe, is to rebuild genuine communities of faith (not communities of certainty). The church or temple will never again be the sole source of authority, but it can be a gathering place of persons who are in search of the Kingdom and are committed to seeing it enacted. I believe that the church has three qualities, which in their combination are nearly unique. First, the church or temple is potentially a place where persons can support and nurture each other. Secondly, it is a place to do the hard work of thinking and organizing for a better world. Third, it is a place to celebrate births, deaths, marriages, healings, and forgiveness.

The route of individualism and self-fulfillment is an empty one in my view. Wholeness emerges out of self-sacrifice more readily than it does out of self-aggrandizement. The religious community gives us a context in which to "die to self" as we commit ourselves to other persons and to a common vision. A great advantage of the religious community over its competitors for allegiance is that it is blessed with heritage and tradition. It can remind the individual that he or she is not the first to face a particular problem or decision. While the past may not be binding, it provides a context for decision-making in a way that those who seek to obliterate history and denigrate community will never realize--to their detriment. In my view, we are only whole when we are in community, supported by the generous arms of a living tradition.

Personally, I find both profound comfort and challenge in the Christian liturgy. I think I might, if born of different parents, have found the same quality in worship as a Jew or Moslem. Not infrequently something stirs deep within me on a Sunday morning. Is it the prayers of confession? Is it the music? Is it the sermon? Is it watching people walk down an aisle to partake in a simple ritual of eating bread and drinking wine--somehow feeling for a moment the equality of all humanity? Or is it the drama of all of these things being orchestrated by a community that is also trying to care for those both within and outside of the community?

Conclusion

Not everyone will find human wholeness in the context of the religious community. Not all religious communities are capable of leading their members into wholeness. For some, salvation will be found in political parties, labor unions, liberation caucuses and other movements where oppression and injustice are deemed the enemy. I doubt whether much wholeness will be found in hot tubs, television-watching, craze diets, and a host of other American obsessions. Whatever the organization or context, however, we have an agenda if we are going to move beyond the superficial appeal of the jargon of wholeness.

Great strides have been made against racism, but the battle is not won. Until it is, the human family cannot be whole. The gap between rich and poor seems to widen rather than recede. Human wholeness is not possible so long as the wealthy defensively guard their assets with guns and power while the poor lust and starve. So long as we are living under the shadow of momentary annihilation by nuclear war, we will not be whole. The psychological numbing that protects us from such an anxiety surely smothers much of our creative energies and capacity for whole-hearted celebration. and what does it mean for us to be constantly threatened by ecological imbalance, environmental pollution, and diminishing resources? When children fear whether they will have the pleasure of a "natural" death, we can surely speculate on the implications for them in achieving human wholeness. Tragically, all of the threats are not so abstract or subtle. What of the "survivors" of bad marriages, underfunded schools, and the barrage of false images of success presented by the media? I must confess my wonder that any flowers bloom in such a wasteland.

References

Bellah, Robert

1964 "Religious Evolution." _American Sociological Review_ 29, 3:358-374.

1967 "Civil Religion in America." _Daedalus_ 96:1-21.

1970 _Beyond Belief: Essays on Religion in a Post-Traditional World_. New York: Harper & Row.

Berger, Peter

1967 _The Sacred Canopy: Elements of a Sociological Theory of Religion_. Garden City, New York: Doubleday.

Berger, Peter, Berger, Brigitte, Kellner, Hansfried

1973 _The Homeless Mind: Modernization and Consciousness_. New York: Random House.

Durkheim, Emile

1964 _The Division of Labor in Society_. Trans. by George Simpson. New York: The Free Press.

1965 _The Elementary Forms of the Religious Life_. Trans. by Joseph Ward Swain. New York: The Free Press.

Freud, Sigmund

1961a _Civilization and Its Discontents_. Trans. & edited by James Strachey. New York: W. W. Norton.

1961b _The Future of an Illusion_. Trans. by W. D. Robson-Scott, revised & edited by James Strachey. Garden City, New York: W. W. Norton.

Herberg, Will

1960 _Protestant-Catholic-Jew: An Essay in American Religious Sociology_. Garden City, New York: Doubleday.

Luckmann, Thomas

1967 The Invisible Religion: The Problem of Religion in Modern Society. London: Macmillan.

Marx, Karl, & Engels, Friedrich

1964 On Religion. Intro. by Reinhold Niebuhr. New York: Schocken.

Miller, Donald

1981 The Case for Liberal Christianity. San Francisco: Harper & Row.

Rhinehart, Luke

1971 The Dice Man. New York: W. Morrow.

Rieff, Phillip

1966 The Triumph of the Therapeutic: Uses of Faith After Freud. New York: Harper & Row.

Weber, Max

1946 From Max Weber: Essays in Sociology. Trans., edited, introd. by H. H. Gerth & C. Wright Mills. New York: Oxford University Press.

1958 The Protestant Ethic and the Spirit of Capitalism. Trans. by Talcott Parsons. New York: Charles Scribner's Sons.

Spirit Centered Wholeness and Education

Nelson L. Haggerson

Focus

The question to be addressed here is, what are the spiritual aspects of individual and societal wholeness from the perspective of Education?

Spirit has many meanings which are found in literature, folklore, religion--making it difficult for an educator to write about spirit in relation to the field of study known as Education, and yet to have taken on the challenge of writing a paper on "spirit-centered wholeness" is a manifestation of my belief in its existence. What I will do in this paper is to write about the phenomenology of spirit in individuals and groups as they are part of the process of education.

In the beginning I will use C. G. Jung's (1982) definition: "spirit is the dynamic principle . . . " Wholeness will mean pervasiveness of both individual and the group (Society). Rather than refer to the entire field of Education, I will confine my discussion to curriculum which is sometimes referred to as the "epistemology" of Education. The "centered" aspect of "spirit-centered wholeness" hinges on the notions of education as distinguished from training, as well as distinguished from instinct, symbols, images and imagination as contrasted with automatic reactions to stimuli.

The Inquiry: A Paradigm for Spirit-Centered Wholeness in Education

How do we educators inquire into the notion of "spirit-centered wholeness"?

Studies of the Person

A number of years ago Carl Rogers and his associates established the Center for Studies of the Person in La Jolla, California. One assumption underlying the creation of this Center was that studies of the person require a much broader, and in some cases basically different, range of research approaches than the "objective scientific" method used and misused by so many researchers. Rogers (1964) conceptualized at least three different methods we might use to study the person: (1) The objective method is one in which the observer makes impartial observations of and experiments with the person(s) being studied and attempts to validate or invalidate those theories. (2) The interpersonal or phenomenological method is one in which the observer is also the observed. Out of the interaction of two persons each comes to know the other and to form tentative theories about the other. These theories can then be tested by asking each other whether the theory was appropriate, by asking a friend or other close observer to confirm the theory, and by observing the actions of the observed to confirm, change, or doubt the theory. (3) The subject method is one in which the person, through self-reflection, theory-making and theory-testing, is both the observer and the observed. Rogers contends that all three of these methods are scientific. Rogers (1964), along with Maslow (1966), Phenix (1975), Kuhn (1970), Lauden (1977), Glaser and

Strauss (1967) and many others, has supported educators in the realization that we needed multiple research methods to study our subjects (persons) and particularly the "dynamic principles" which seem to underlie their behaviors and actions. Furthermore, they have given us suggestions such as those referred to above and attributed to Rogers.

Studies of Societies

In addition to realizing the need for research methods and modes of inquiry with which to study individual persons, we have discovered that our classrooms are mini-societies and that the anthropologists who have been studying societies for years have much to offer us in the form of ethnographic methods (Wolcott, 1982). We have been aware of the spirit (dynamic principle) of the classroom for a long time, but we have needed the ethnographic research emphasis to allow us to inquire more deeply into the phenomenology of spirit in the classroom.

Studies of Content

Besides studies of the person (individual) and studies of classrooms as small societies, educators need to know the nature of textual materials, learning events, metaphors, symbols and language, all of which are integral parts of our domain. There seems to be a spirit (dynamic principle) underlying these aspects of education, too. Many of us have had a poem or piece of literature, a painting or symbol, a fairy tale or a myth, literally speak to us. But how do we study the phenomenology of the spirit of a text? Palmer (1967) and Ricoeur (1981) among others have given us a rationale for adapting and using the hermeneutic or hermeneutic-historical methods of inquiry with which to interpet texts and events.

Naturalistic Research Paradigms

The research methods mentioned above are all what we are now calling "Naturalistic" methods, and they are part of a large tradition of inquiry which is called a "Naturalistic Research Paradigm" (Belok and Haggerson, 1982). They give a basis from which to inquire about the phenomenology of spirit as it relates to education (curriculum). It is inquiry within this naturalistic research paradigm that has guided me to spirit-centered wholeness.

The objectives of research done within the naturalistic paradigm are called, among other things, "naturalistic generalizations" (Stake and Trumbull). A naturalistic generalization evokes a vicarious experience on the part of the reader of the research. That is, the researcher does the research and reports. The reader reads the report and says, "Oh, yes, I understand that," or the reader has a joyful experience when reading the report, or the reader recoils when reading the report. These are all manifestations of vicarious experiences when the reader identifies with the research report. The form and the substance of the research report, then, are both important. A research report might be in the form of a poem, a song, a vignette, a short story, a formal statement, or a theory.

What else does explication of the naturalistic research paradigm, its methods and its objectives, contribute to Spirit-Centered Wholeness in Education? Over the years educators have avoided reference to "spirit" and certainly any research relating to "spirit" for two reasons (at least): in the first place, spirit has been linked to religion, and so the separation of church and state stipulation of the Constitution has kept us from inquiry. Secondly, the predominant research paradigm in education has been the "scientific/objective" one. It has focused on behavior, traits, parts, and status aspects of curriculum and methods. On the other hand, the naturalistic research paradigm is concerned with the "whole," with relationships, with dynamics, with interpersonal phenomena, with subjective phenomena and their conceptualization. In that sense it contributes to our inquiring about what holds us together, what are the vitality and regenerating qualities which survive the changes culture--hence the notion of spirit. The fact that we are researching what I call in this paper the phenomenology of spirit by methods that are available to all may allay the concerns of those who might charge that we are mixing religion with the schools (violating separation of church and state in the case of public schools).

Finally, in employing naturalistic research methods we may join other communities of scholars in the basic objective of hermeneutics: "The basic aim is grasping the 'spirit of antiquity,' which is most clearly revealed in the literary heritage." We want to join those, too, who are searching for the "spirit of today and tomorrow."

Categories of Spirit-Centered Wholeness

Two of the main aspects of an academic discipline or a professional field of study are methods of inquiry (syntax) and conceptualizations, generalizations, theories and facts (substantive dimension). I have just discussed some forms of inquiry used in education which might render concepts, categories, and theories about spirit-centered wholeness. Now I will discuss some of those substantive components.

Glaser and Strauss (1967) write about arranging data into categories. The final arrangement focuses on what they call "core" categories around which other categories of data cluster. As I have examined the data, I see them centering around spiritual aspects of individuals, groups, and curriculum content which I call core categories. In the following sections I will discuss each of these categories. Later, in the theory section, I will show the relatedness of these categories, hence demonstrating "wholeness" (pervasiveness of spirit).

Curriculum Content

At first blush it may seem odd to think of curriculum content as spirit-centered. However, when we think of not only the areas of curriculum content (humanities, sciences, mathematics, history, languages, health sciences . . .) but also the nature of the content within those areas (concepts, images, symbols, signs, metaphors, epochs, cycles, sounds, patterns, myths, fairy tales . . .), we may get a glimpse of spirit-centered curriculum content.

Literature. For instance, consider with Jung (1982) the spirit motif as it appears in fairy tales:

> The frequency with which the spirit types appear as an old man is about the same in fairy tales as in dreams. The old man always appears when the hero is in a hopeless and desperate situation from which only profound reflection or a happy idea--in other words, a spiritual function or an endo-

> psychic automatism of some kind--can extricate him. But since, for internal and external reasons, the hero cannot accomplish this himself, the knowledge needed to compensate the deficiency comes in the form of a personified thought, i.e., in the shape of this sagacious and helpful old man. (p. 13)

The reader (learner) of this fairy tale can easily see that "the old man represents knowledge, reflection, wisdom, cleverness and intuition on the one hand, and on the other, moral qualities such as goodwill and readiness to help, which make its 'spiritual' character sufficiently plain" (p. 17).

I recently presented a paper at the Fourth Annual Conference on Curriculum Theorizing entitled "Reconceptualizing Professional Literature: An Aesthetic Study" (Haggerson, 1982) in which I interpreted and reinterpreted three pieces of literature by using the "hermeneutic spiral." The method was an adaption of the hermeneutic circle used by Ast and Dilthey (Palmer, 1969). This research process led to several naturalistic generalizations: Using the hermeneutic spiral brings out much of one's own experiential background. It also helps one move out of the isolation of "individuality" and toward the realization that each of us is an inseparable part of the universe. There is a discernible relationship between the writer, the critic, the reader, the piece of literature, and the hermeneutic process of interpretation. As the writer of "The Box Thing" (and others), I did not know the piece contained so much meaning. As a critic I found more than I had as an author. As a reader (reading out loud to others) I found aspects of the poem that I didn't find as a writer or critic. As a listener to the responses of others, as well as a reader of their written responses, I discovered still other dimensions of the opus. It behooves us as writers, readers, and critics of literature to try on different roles, to let the hermeneutic spiral work in that way, too. I concluded with Dilthey (Palmer, 1969) that "A piece of literature is a form of spiritual nourishment which brings to expression other wellsprings of the life in which we move" (p. 122).

A naturalistic generalization in the form of a poem describes the naturalistic writer:

The Sculpture

(The Naturalistic Writer)

The artist walking by
Picked up a lump of clay
and moistened it.
With fingers warm he smoothed,
Plucked, shaped and urged
His life into the form.
Spirit for his spirit
Danced in clay.
It caught the music
Of his heart, and breathed.

(Dorothy Lykes in Haggerson, 1971)

The point here is to emphasize that literature, be it in the form of fairy tales, professional writing, plays, short stories, when interpreted via hermeneutics, seems to have a "spiritual" autonomy of its own. That spirit transcends time and space--the classics are eternal--it transcends cultures and countries. Furthermore, literature is the manifestation of images, metaphor, and ideas created by humans and yet once created it stands autonomously. As Gadamer (Palmer, 1969) said, "the literary piece having been created speaks to its critics, readers and listeners."

Science. Manifestations of the "spiritual" aspects of curriculum content, similar to those in literature, can be found in Science (Shrodinger, 1982), Psychology (Jung, 1982; Hillman, 1975), and History (Kaegi, 1982).

The Individual (Person)

Self. One aspect of the spiritual individual is what we call the self. The self is written about in sociological, psychological, philosophical, religious and educational literature. One principle that is explored by Combs (1961) in the books entitled Perceiving, Behaving, Becoming, and Individual Behavior (Combs & Snygg, 1959) is that an individual's behavior is determined by one's attempts to gain and maintain an acceptable self-concept. This view is not held by all educators or psychologists. B. F. Skinner (1953), in his book Science and Human Behavior, tries to convince us that reinforced behavior is the essential component of an individual's motivation, that such invisibles as self, freedom and dignity are hindrances to human progress. My experience as teacher, parent, learner, person and researcher leads me to conclude, with Combs, that there is a spiritual dimension underlying behavior, whether or not we call it "self."

Controlled patterns. Zoologist Adolf Portmann (1982) speaks of the "phenomena in which the spiritual is manifested" as "inwardness," "playfulness," "representational value of forms" (the meanings humans put on external organs), and controlled patterns which are called "civilized." He concludes his discussion of spirit by saying, 'Spiritual' means here the special activity of man which creates the instrument of controlled expression, and which helps him to master his peculiar existence" (p. 368).

Transcendence. Our ability to transcend time and space and to have vicarious experiences are other manifestations of the spiritual nature of an individual. Phenix (1975) talks about these human characteristics as "transcendence in the curriculum." If we didn't have the spiritual ability to transcend, our curriculum content of words, concepts, images, symbols would be meaningless, and we would be confined to firsthand experience for all learning. Jung (1982) put it this way:

> The hallmarks of spirit are, firstly, the principle of spontaneous movement and activity; secondly, the spontaneous capacity to produce images independently of sense perception; and thirdly, the autonomous and sovereign manipulation of these images. (p. 88)

Archetypes. Jung (1968) uses the terms "archetype" and "collective unconscious" to refer to the dynamic principle, spirit. One set of archetypes which seem pertinent here are those which undergird personality types. Jung (1971) and many of his followers indicate that each of us has a tendency toward behaving and seeing the world in certain ways. These tendencies are personality functions. We tend to be "introverted" or "extroverted," "intuitive" or "sensing," "thinking" or "feeling." These functions are sufficiently distinguishable to permit the development of instruments (surveys) with which to "measure" them. The Myers-Briggs and the Gray-Wheelright instruments are examples. The unfortunate thing that happens is that some identify the score on the survey instrument with the reality and tend to stereotype people into narrow categories. The point to be made here is that the archetypes are pervasive (universal) and spiritual. They manifest themselves in the tendencies and actions of human beings.

The individual person, then, seems to have "spirit" as the basis of "self," "inwardness," "playfulness," "representational value of forms," "controlled patterns of the civilized," "spontaneous movement and activity," "spontaneous capacity to produce images independently of sense perceptions," "autonomous and sovereign manipulation of these images," "transcendence" and "personality types," to mention the ones discussed in this section of the paper.

The individual is surely a vital part of the educational process and knowledge of the individual person is necessary for us educators to engage in our field of study, Education. However, individuals are also social beings, they are part of a classroom, they are part of a group. So the next challenge is to explore the "spirit-centered wholeness" of the group (society).

The Group

Esprit de corps. We have probably all experienced phenomena within a group of people which we called *esprit de corps*. I have surely experienced it, as have students in my classes. Recently I met a person who had been in a class of 42 people 20 years ago. He said, "Do you remember that class? I can still feel the *esprit de corps*. I can still remember how energized I was every week when I left class. I have forgotten a lot of classroom experiences, but I will never forget that one." So the *esprit de corps* phenomena seem to affect memory, to generate energy, stimulate learning, and recreate emotion when one is remembering the group. It implies people working together, "resonating" and having good feelings about one another. In an article entitled, "Listen to Learning," Garman (1980) and I describe classrooms which manifest the <u>esprit de corps</u>. We say they become "organic" (interrelated) classrooms or groups. The organic classroom generates its own content, its own rules of order, its own outcomes; class members relate to one another in what might be called "synergistic" ways.

<u>Synergy</u>. Synergy is the phenomenon described by the principle, "the whole is greater than the sum of its parts." The term "synergy" seems to have been applied to groups or societies first by anthropologist Ruth Benedict (Bartell, 1982). Benedict used "high synergy" to describe those societies whose members were observed to enhance each other. One member's achievement enhanced other members. In a society of "low synergy" one member, in order to achieve, would diminish another member. We sometimes say, "in order to get ahead one has to step on another." The organic classroom is one of high synergy.

Bartell (1982) did a study with synergistic couples in which she discovered that their behaviors, attitudes, and relationships were often polar and always dynamic. For instance, within a synergistic couple there was playfulness and seriousness, masculinity and femininity--and those attributes were often manifested first by one member of the couple, and then by the other. Garman and I recognized these relationships in our organic classroom.

<u>Metaphor</u>. Another aspect of the synergistic couple study and the organic classroom is the aesthetic. Bartell reports her aesthetic experiences

in conducting the research. Garman and I also had aesthetic experiences in conducting the research. While we are able to describe our experiences fairly well and while we have some explanations for the phenomena, we ultimately resort to a metaphorical statement such as, "The whole is greater than the sum of its parts," or "The esprit de corps of the classroom is remarkable!" We all seem to be exploring the phenomenology of "spirit-centered wholeness," and most often use metaphor to describe ourselves.

Patriotism, friendship and loves. After World War II some studies were done to try to explain patriotism among soldiers. One conclusion of the studies was that the binding force which allowed soldiers (marines, sailors) to sacrifice was "friendship." What the studies didn't do was explain friendship. Similar studies to explain love have fallen into the same limitations. We experience love among people as caring, helping, sexual, romantic, survival, and yet we are only able to grapple with phenomena, not the spirit of love.

Groups of people, classrooms of students, assemblies of patriots, rallies of youths . . . (society), too, seem to be characterized by "spirit-centered wholeness." The size of the group doesn't seem to be sufficient explanation for its spirituality or wholeness, nor does the location or the purpose. And yet, as the student of 20 years ago, we know, sense, feel, experience it, the dynamic principle, the spirit, the wholeness, the esprit de corps, and the synergy.

Spirit of search. As scientists, educators, or researchers in various disciplines, we may find ourselves with Adolf Portmann (1982), the biologist:

> For no one can define the limits of human investigation, nor even of biology, when it seeks know-

> ledge of the spiritual. But to realize and keep constantly in mind that there are limits, even when we cannot measure their proximity or remoteness, is one of the prerequisites of the scientific attitude. (p. 330)

We might even say, "The spirit of the scientific attitude, or the spirit of a community of scholars."

The Theory

Spirit-Centered Wholeness in Education

The poem "Oneness" was written after I had a profound experience, a spiritual experience; it represents the quintessence of my theory.

Oneness

The oneness of it all is
A house of many mansions,
Multiple levels of consciousness,
Infinite individual personalities . . .
Juxtaposed in dynamic relationships
  called a
  Universe.

(Haggerson, 1974)

The relationships between/within curriculum content, individuals, and groups are wholistic; they are spiritual. The contents of the curriculum depend on individuals or groups who create them, yet once they are created they have an autonomy of their own; they spark individuals and groups to create other content, to form other images, metaphors; they foster other dynamic relationships. The classroom (group or society) is more than the sum of its parts; it is synergistic. It, too, is created by/for individuals, yet its *esprit de corps* gives it an integrity of its own. The individual person has a spiritual aspect, too. That spiritual property of the individual transcends time and space; it is the "principle of spontaneous movement and activity, of the spontaneous capacity to produce images independently of sense perceptions, and the autonomous and sovereign manipulation of those images." The spiritual quality of the relationship permits idealization of and motivation toward the oneness of it all.

Implications for Curriculum (Education)

As implied in the preceding sections, an awareness of the essential nature of the individual, the group and the content of the curriculum is necessary if one is to understand the spiritual aspect of education. This necessity further implies that we create an educational environment (Roberts, 1975) which fosters study to create awareness; that we develop and teach appropriate methods of inquiry and research, that we develop and teach attitudes and skills which foster dialogue and discussion about the significant aspects of individuals, groups and content; that we develop, teach, and model dispositions which contribute to the understanding of "spirit-centered wholeness," some of which are "hope, faith, wonder, awe, reverence, concern for wholeness, doubt, criticism and creativity" (Phenix, 1975). The universality of spirit implies that a curriculum to cultivate its understanding is for all students, not just for gifted ones. The history of the phenomenology of spirit is fraught with conflict and contradictions, hence a curriculum concerned with its understanding must promote, besides attitudes of hope and criticism and skills of inquiry and questioning, patience, patience for learning and inquiring about the infinite. Finally the attitude and value of idealization should be fostered. Idealizations (perfection) can be stifling, but put in proper perspective they are motivating. These implications themselves are an idealization. Hopefully, like the curriculum content written about earlier, they will speak to us.

References

Bartell, S. In Support of Grounded Theory: One Researcher's Experience. Review Journal of Philosophy and Social Science, 1982, 7 (1 and 2).

Belok, M., & Haggerson, N. L. Naturalistic Research Paradigms. Meerut, India: ANU Books, 1982.

Campbell, J. (Ed.). Spirit and Nature: Papers From the Eranos Yearbooks, Bollingen Series XXX-1. First Princeton/Bollingen Paperback printing. Princeton: Princeton University Press, 1982.

Combs, A. W. (Ed.). Perceiving, Behaving, Becoming. Washington, D.C.: Association for Supervision and Curriculum Development, 1962.

Combs, A. W., & Snygg, D. Individual Behavior: A Perceptual Approach. New York: Harper, 1959.

Froebe-Kaptezn, O. Preface. In J. Campbell (Ed.). Spirit and Nature: Papers From the Eranos Yearbooks, Bollingen Series XXX-1. First Princeton/Bollingen Paperback printing. Princeton: Princeton University Press, 1982.

Garman, N., & Haggerson, N. L. Listen to the Learning: Toward a Pedagogy for Philosophy of Education. In M. Belok and J. L. Green (Eds.), Philosophy and Education. Meerut, India: ANU Praxashan, 1980.

Glaser, B. G., & Strauss, A. L. The Discovery of Grounded Theory: Strategies for Qualitative Research. New York: Aldine Publishing, 1967.

Haggerson, N. L. To Dance With Joy. Jericho, NY: Exposition Press, 1971.

Haggerson, N. L. Oneness. In G. Sargent (Ed.). The Other Poetry Book. Bigfork, MN: Northwoods Press, 1974.

Haggerson, N. L. Reconceptualizing Professional Literature: An Aesthetic Self Study. A paper presented at the Fourth Conference on Curriculum Theory and Practice, Warrenton, VA, 1982.

Hillman, J. Re-visioning Psychology. New York: Harper and Row, 1975.

Jung, C. G. The Archetypes and the Collective Unconscious (2nd ed.). Princeton: Princeton University Press, 1968.

Jung, C. G. Psychological Types (2nd. ed.). Princeton: Princeton University Press, 1971.

Jung, C. G. The Phenomenology of Spirit. In J. Campbell (Ed.), Spirit and nature: Papers From the Eranos Yearbooks, Bollingen Series XXX-1. First Princeton/Bollingen Paperback printing. Princeton: Princeton University Press, 1982.

Jung, C. G. The Spirit of Psychology. In J. Campbell (Ed.), Spirit and Nature: Papers From the Eranos Yearbooks, Bollingen Series XXX-1. First Princeton/Bollingen Paperback printing. Princeton University Press, 1982.

Kaegi, W. The Transformation of the Spirit in the Renaissance. In J. Campbell (Ed.), Spirit and Nature: Papers From the Eranos Yearbooks, Bollingen Series XXX-1. First Princeton/Bollingen Paperback printing. Princeton: Princeton University Press, 1982.

Kuhn, T. S. The Structure of Scientific Revolutions. International Encyclopedia of Unified Science, 1970, 11, (2).

Laudan, L. Progress and its Problems: Towards a Theory of Scientific Growth. Berkeley: University of California Press, 1977.

Maslow, A. H. The Psychology of Science. Chicago: Henry Regnery Co., 1966.

Palmer, R. E. Hermeneutics: Interpretation Theory in Schleiermacher, Dilthey, Heidegger, and Gadamer. Evanston, IL: Northwestern University Press, 1969.

Phenix, P. Transcendence in the Curriculum. In Pinar (Ed.), Curriculum Theorizing: The Reconceptualists. Berkeley: McCutchan Publishing, 1975.

Portmann, A. Biology and the Phenomenon of the Spiritual. In J. Campbell (Ed.), Spirit and Nature: Papers From the Eranos Yearbooks, Bollingen Series XXX-1. First Princeton/Bollingen Paperback printing. Princeton: Princeton University Press, 1982.

Ricoeur, P. Hermeneutics and the Human Sciences. Cambridge: Cambridge University Press, 1981.

Roberts, T. B. Four Psychologies Applied to Education: Freudian, Behavioral, Humanistic and Transpersonal. New York: John Wiley & Sons, 1975.

Rogers, C. Toward a Science of the Person. In T. W. Wann (Ed.). Behaviorism and Phenomenology. Chicago: University of Chicago Press, 1964.

Schrodinger, E. The Spirit of Science. In J. Campbell (Ed.), Spirit and Nature: Papers From the Eranos Yearbooks. Bollingen Series XXX-1. First Princeton/Bollingen Paperback printing. Princeton: Princeton University Press, 1982.

Skinner, B. F. Science and Human Behavior. New York: Macmillan Company, 1953.

Stake, R. E., & Trumbull, D. J. Naturalistic Generalizations. In M. Belok and N. L. Haggerson, (Eds.), Naturalistic Research Paradigm. Meerut, India: ANU Press, 1982.

Wilbur, K. (Ed.). The Holograph Paradigm and Other Paradoxes. Boulder: Shambhala, 1982.

Wolcott, H. F. Differing Styles of On-site Research, or If it isn't Ethnography, What is it? Review Journal of Philosophy and Social Science, 1982, 7 (1 and 2).

SPIRITUAL WHOLENESS

Wholeness Centered in Spirit

John B. Cobb, Jr.

"Wholeness" and "spirit" have diverse meaning. This paper describes two ideals for human existence associated respectively with selected meanings. Understood in this way spirit as commitment to a transcending cause is in tension with wholeness. Wholeness cannot be expanded to include spirit, but if the cause to which spirit is committed is sufficiently inclusive, spirit-centered wholeness is possible. Such a wholeness lacks the spontaneity of wholeness without spirit. This spontaneity can be recovered in wholeness centered in spirit.

Introduction

In recent reflections about the ideal for human existence, the language of wholeness and the language of spirit rarely go together. They connote quite different ideals in considerable tension with each other. To formulate the ideal of wholeness centering in spirit is to introduce the tension into the ideal itself. This provokes fresh reflection on the meanings of the key terms and on the nature of the human ideal.

This paper is written from the perspective of a Christian theologian. Theologians have spoken more of "spirit" than of "wholeness." Indeed, the heroes of the Christian tradition are not noted for their "wholeness." Yet "wholeness" belongs to a family of words, including holiness, that have played a very prominent role in Christian history. And Christians who have largely lost the ability to think in terms of holiness have found the new ideas of holiness as wholeness, coming from humanistic psychology, appealing, if also somehow troubling.

The terms "spirit" and "wholeness" are both fluid in their meaning and use. In theology, also, there are diverse uses of these terms. There would be no difficulty in so defining them that the tensions they introduce would vanish, but little would be gained by such a procedure. I propose instead to present brief pictures of two human ideals. I associate one with wholeness, the other with spirit. Although I do not assert that others must have the same ideals in mind when they use these terms, I hope my use will not seem eccentric. It will be clear from these accounts that wholeness and spirit in these senses cannot be simply merged. That will pose the question as to whether there is another kind of wholeness which can center in spirit. I will argue that there is, and will offer a brief account of spirit-centered wholeness.

What will thereby be depicted, however, remains unsatisfactory. This spirit-centered wholeness lacks the attractive spontaneity and presence of the wholeness which is indifferent to spirit. The final proposal of the paper is that for the renewal of spontaneity without loss of spirit, we must move from spirit-centered wholeness to Spirit-centered wholeness.

1. The ideal of wholeness

There are many ideas of what human existence ideally should be. One of the most prominent, one which has seemed self-evident to many, is that of ethical righteousness. It seems that people should do in every instance what they should do. The problem of defining the ideal, then, is the problem of identifying the norms, rules, principles, or virtues by which this obligation is determined. The problem of realizing the ideal is the problem of overcoming inward resistance to the requirements of these norms. Those who advocate the ideas connoted by wholeness and by spirit reject the ethical one as too limited. They do not, of course, propose that violation of ethical norms is desirable. But they believe that the life that centers in the effort to be righteous is inadequate and unsatisfactory.

The most thorough and influential theological discussion of the alternative ideals for human existence has been that of Søren Kierkegaard. He distinguished the aesthetic, the ethical, and the religious as the three great options. He identified them as stages with a clear sense that the movement of progress was from aesthetic to the ethical and from the ethical to the religious. If the Christian imposes this scheme on the alternatives now before us, the quest for wholeness will seem to be at the aesthetic stage, and the ideal of spirit at the religious. We could then suppose that the two alternatives to ethical righteousness are sub-ethical on the one side and supra-ethical on the other.

Such an analysis is not irrelevant to the contemporary scene. Some of the same psychological developments that have led to the ideal of wholeness have led also to the glorification of what SK described as the aesthetic. Some of those who seek wholeness are aware of the inadequacy of this sub-ethical response. They seek a mode of existence that will incorporate what is necessary and desirable in ethical conduct in a wider context. In that context what truly conforms to ethical righteousness will be done as an expression of what one is rather than in opposition to one's continuing desires. This draws aside attention to rules and principles, but it encourages relationships with others which will attain the ends sought by conformity to such rules and principles more effectively than does the preoccupation with ethical righteousness. In these ways it resembles SK's religious stage more than the aesthetic. It may be better understood as an alternative form of the religious than a falling back to the aesthetic.

What is this alternative to the ideal of ethical righteousness which can be named as "wholeness"? It is, first, a rejection of dualism. The life lived according to the ethical ideal is inevitably dualistic. One tries to do what is right even when one does not want to do it. One experiences resistance to the right within oneself. In terms of the ethical ideal the sources of this resistance are necessarily viewed as evil. One ought to be faithful to one's spouse. One desires another. That desire is evil and when one acts upon it, that is a sin. The will to overcome that desire and act righteously is good.

There is today a great deal of psychological wisdom pointing to the negative consequences of this dualism. The desire labeled evil does not go away, and the moral struggle against it leads to a preoccupation with illicit sexuality. There is a strong tendency to envy those who actually, or in the fantasy of the righteous, give way to temptation, and to desire their punishment because of this envy. There is also a strong tendency to blame others for the power of evil within oneself--witness the extensive blaming of women for the sins of men. If, on the other hand, one yields to temptation, this is followed or accompanied by intense feelings of guilt which may not prevent repetition of the sin but which do have destructive consequences for the personality as a whole. These complex dynamics are today well-known and do not require elaboration here.

The ideal to which I am pointing by "wholeness" rejects this dualism of right and wrong, good and evil, will and desire. It accepts human reality as it is with all of its wants and desires. It condemns nothing. It affirms that precisely when nothing is condemned, nothing becomes destructive. All one's impulses can be acknowledged and accepted for what they are. They should be viewed hierarchically as if some were more noble than others. Each is what it is and has its rightful place in the whole. Sexuality is to be accepted and enjoyed as a pervasive aspect of life without guilt about that expression. In general a mark of wholeness is freedom from compulsiveness and legalistic rules.

What I am calling human wholeness in its ideal form is not found apart from relationships. Indeed, it is experienced and lived only in relationships. Thus, those who are whole persons accept the whole range of emotions within themselves and can be themselves with others and allow others to be themselves as well. This does not make for trouble-free relationships. But it makes for authenticity, depth, genuine sharing, spontaneity, and growth. Whole persons can sustain long-term relationships, but they can also accept their rupture.

Those who are whole can enjoy others, but they have no need for the constant company of others. They do not need the admiration or affection of others as a basis for acceptance of themselves. Hence they have no general need to please others or to win success or fame. They enjoy relationships with the world of non-human creatures as well as with human beings, and they can enjoy times of being alone with their own thoughts and feelings. They can appreciate beauty, but they have no compulsion to attain refined aesthetic tastes. They can enjoy being creative, but they have no need to demonstrate their gifts to themselves or to others. They are adventurous and curious, but they do not have to pile novelty upon novelty to avoid boredom.

Perhaps the central image for "whole" persons is "at-homeness." They are "at-home" in their bodies, in their conscious and unconscious feelings and senses, in their human relationships, and in their total natural environment. They are "at-home" with who they are, and therefore they are comfortable being just that.

Because they are "at-home" in themselves, they are free from defensiveness toward others. Others experience their warmth--that is their openness, their concern, and their affection. One is not the object of good deeds or just treatment from the whole person. One is the recipient of acceptance and understanding.

2. The ideal of Spirit

The ideal associated with spirit is a quite different alternative to the limitations of ethical righteousness. The ethical person attempts to make each decision rightly. The spiritual person is captured by a vision of what is needful or desirable and is dedicated to its service or realization. What is to be done is ordered by the convictions which the vision expresses and the commitments that follow from it. The vision may take innumerable forms. For example, it may be of a people freed from oppression, or of a world in which peace is secure, or of a society in which the fulfillment of each conduces to the fulfillment of all. It may combine such elements as these in a larger whole.

Persons of spirit in this sense live from and for visions such as these. This means that their personal fulfillment is subordinated to wider purposes. There is no inherent value in self-sacrifice, but when the larger good can be realized only through actions that are personally costly, these actions, including the laying down of one's life, will be taken.

Personal morality will also be relativized. The need to be morally pure, characteristic of the ethical life, is set aside. This does not mean that conformity to generally accepted ethical principles will be lightly ignored. But for the realization of the larger purposes, one's self-image as a righteous person may have to be sacrificed.

Relationships with others are important for spiritual persons. But these are not ends in themselves simply to be enjoyed or to be valued as means to personal growth. Relationships subserve the cause. It is precisely in shared commitment to that which is beyond themselves and beyond the relationships that the relationships attain their full meaning and depth.

Our psychological culture encourages the suspicion that those who commit themselves to overriding causes do so out of an emotional need. For example, one's need to be approved by others and by oneself may lead to dramatic acts of sacrifice. There is no doubt that "causes" attract people who have such psychological needs, often unhealthy ones. But if it is true that no one is committed to work for world peace because world peace is truly important and desirable, more important and desirable than personal satisfactions and enjoyments, then the idea of spirit is an illusion. The assumption of this paper is that spirit is just as real as emotion. That does not mean that there would be people of spirit whose convictions and commitments are free of emotional concomitants. Indeed, in the real world I assume that there are distorting aspects in these emotional concomitants in all cases. The ideal associated with spirit, however, is that these concomitants distort, and such distortion is sufficiently a matter of degree that we can understand the ideal of its elimination.

Persons who are genuinely and purely committed to inclusive purposes tend to experience the many aspects of their own personal existence with a certain detachment. Their identity is bound up with the service of the cause. This does not make their bodily and emotional needs disappear. To some extent these can be correlated with the service of the cause, but for the most part some tension remains between emotion and spirit.

According to this ideal, people of spirit will not view this tension in dualistic terms as coming from evil and expressing itself in sin. If they speak of evil and sin, as they may well do, it will be in terms of the great social forces that make for oppression and war. But they know that in the process of serving the cause they must deal with those aspects of their own makeup which make claims on them discontinuous with that service. How they do that varies greatly. Gandhi's choice of celibacy and sexual sublimation is one example. Others may choose a mode of alternation in which periods of ascetic devotion to the cause are balanced by others in which bodily and emotional needs are cared for. As another possibility we will consider later the ideal of wholeness centering in spirit. What is common to all of these is a conscious and reflective decision as to how to deal with the various aspects of one's personal existence.

Spiritual persons have great power over others. The unification of their lives and energies around a cause attracts others to that cause and to them as leaders. Justifications for narrower foci of life and primary attention to personal interests are shattered by contact with spiritual people. They are not comfortable to be around. They force decisions that most people do not want to make. But they fascinate as well as repel, and their words have authority.

The ideal of persons of spirit is of persons who are free from the need to be approved or liked. If they desire success, it is because their success is conducive to that of the cause. If they desire fame, it is because visibility and reputation enable them to increase their contribution to the cause.

3. The combination of wholeness and Spirit

Among the many possible ideals for human existence I have sketched two, which I have distinguished with these words "wholeness" and "spirit." They are presented, of course, as ideals, not as descriptions of actual people. Nevertheless, they are not remote and unrealizable ideals. There are persons who approximate wholeness, and there are others who approximate spirit. Although most of us are far from embodying either ideal, to subscribe to one or the other is likely to exercise considerable influence in our lives.

The suggestion of the topic of this conference is that many of us find attractiveness in both ideals and desire in some way to combine them. The fact that we are holding such a conference also indicates that such a combination is not a simple matter.

The problem appears most clearly when we begin with wholeness. It may seem that the need would be simply to expand wholeness to include more and more, in this case, spirit. But when approached from this side we find a double meaning in "wholeness." One idea is that of inclusiveness, the other, that of completeness and self-containedness. These are in tension. The ideal of wholeness I have sketched is dominated by the latter. It is, of course, inclusive of a great deal, but it is not inclusive of everything. Specifically, it is not inclusive of spirit. If it attempts to include spirit, it loses its completeness and self-containedness. It would not be expanded, it would be radically altered.

This is because this ideal of wholeness is realized by the rejection of heteronomous requirements laid upon oneself from beyond the self. The rejection is primarily of ethical requirements, but it must include those of the spirit as well. The non-hierarchical appreciation of all aspects of human existence is incompatible with ordering them to a purpose which transcends personal existence. This does not mean that the attainment of this ideal of wholeness excludes contributing to good causes. It does not. But these contributions must be expressions of concerns that arise non-hierarchically alongside other concerns. They cannot be all-consuming.

If wholeness and spirit cannot be brought together by an expansion of wholeness, can they be united from the side of spirit? The difficulties on this side are enormous. If, as we are likely to agree, Gandhi is a great spiritual leader of our century who comes as close as anyone to embodying the ideal of spirit, we will also agree that he did not embody the ideal of wholeness. For the sake of India and the world, he not only repressed or sublimated his sexuality; he also abused his body with extreme fasting. His emotional life and personal relationships, including those with his children, also suffered from his commitment to Indian independence. In these respects he is not untypical of spiritual leaders. For example, it is saddening to observe the cost to self and family paid by many of the leaders in the struggle against the Vietnam War. In many cultures it has been held that the ideal of spirit cannot mix with family life. The ideal of a wholeness centering in spirit, therefore, is in sharp contrast with the dominant ideals associated with spirit and with their major approximations in history.

Nevertheless, the remainder of this paper will deal with the ideal of spirit-centered wholeness. The intention is not that this ideal displace all existing ideals including those of wholeness and of spirit. At least at our present juncture we need a plurality of ideals. But for those such as myself who cannot abandon the ideal of spirit, who see it indeed as particularly needful in a time when catastrophe threatens all, but who are distressed by its historic role of denial of personal wholeness, the ideal of spirit-centered wholeness has importance and even urgency.

4. The possibility and limitations of spirit-centered wholeness

Characteristic of people of spirit is the critical objectification of the various aspects of their own being. They reflect about their sexuality and their human relationships, for example, in light of their convictions and commitments. This does not itself conduce to wholeness. On the contrary, the ordering of these aspects of their lives to purposes that are alien to them more generally leads to sacrifices or to unintegrated alternations. To order one's life to the liberation of a people from political oppression probably necessitates the rejection of wholeness.

This follows from the fact that although the vision that controls commitment and conviction is a very large one, it is not itself inclusive. Those devoted to the liberation of a particular people from a particular oppression usually know that there are other needs in the world as well. But these other needs often do not constitute an effective part of their vision. Hence they order their whole lives to the limited goal. This cannot be integrative of all aspects of their personal being.

The situation is only a little improved if they do concern themselves with the political liberation of all oppressed people. This has the advantage of relativizing the needs of one people and therefore reducing the likelihood that the liberation of one group will be at the expense of others. But with respect to the dimensions of personal experience, little is changed. All will be ordered to political ends.

The situation is changed, however, if the vision which shapes convictions and commitments is of a whole world of whole people. In this vision it is clear that freedom from war and political oppression cannot be separated from the wholeness of personal life and personal relationships. The ordering of all aspects of one's existence to this goal will ideally involve their positive inclusion in an integrated form. In practice, of course, compromises are required. For the sake of the wholeness of all, some may have to sacrifice their wholeness and even their lives. But in this vision it is recognized that the failure to attain to personal wholeness is a failure to contribute to the realization of the vision just as much as it is a failure to alter public structures.

This account is very formal and abstract. It would seem nearly irrelevant to the real historical situation if it were not for the effective existence of the feminist movement. In that movement the unity of the personal and the political is being increasingly recognized in theory and realized in practice. This points to the meaningfulness and worthwhileness of proposing the ideal of spirit-centered wholeness.

A complete account of the ideal of spirit-centered wholeness would be impossible and even undesirable. But illustrations of how it is already being expressed will help to give some concreteness to the otherwise disembodied ideal. For some people of spirit the all-determining cause is that of preventing massive starvation and providing food for the world's hungry. The study of the cause and cures of the global food problem will lead to complex answers, but one among the causes will be the excessive consumption of meat, and especially beef, in affluent cultures. A natural response will be to reduce, if not eliminate, meat consumption. This response may be made by a spiritual person even at some risk to personal health.

If, however, the spiritual person orients life to a more inclusive vision, the personal embodiment of physical health will appear not only as a private desideration that should be readily sacrificed to a larger cause but as a part of what is globally desirable. At the same time, it will not be assumed that there must be a trade-off between eating for one's personal health and eating in a way that is appropriate to the concern for world hunger. On the contrary, one will look for ways of eating that are appropriate to both at once. Once the question is posed in this way it is not hard to find answers. Indeed, on the whole, the kind of eating that is inappropriate to a world of scarcity is also unhealthful for individuals, and the kind of eating that is good for individuals would be compatible with meeting the need for food of all people. The book, Diet for a Small Planet, expresses the unity of these concerns.

In other respects such synergistic solutions are more difficult and complex. As long as we live in Southern California we find ourselves forced to choose between an immobility that would be personally and socially costly and involvement in a system of transportation that is outrageously expensive in terms of the resources of the world, appallingly destructive of our own environment and alarmingly harmful to our health. We can buy smaller and more efficient cars and drive at more efficient speeds. But these are minor compromises rather than basic responses. Caught within the established system no life-style is possible that is appropriate to the inclusive vision.

The alternative is first to conceive and then to create a different context for human living. This is not impossible. Paolo Soleri is far in advance in conceiving this different form of human habitat, and he is doing what he can to build an experimental model.

Soleri's city would simultaneously be far more frugal with respect to the earth's resource and far more humanizing in social relationships. It would restore the aesthetic dimension to our public lives and make our environment more healthful. If Soleri's cities were actually built they could embody much of what we mean by spirit-centered wholeness. The general apathy toward his experiment is an indication of how little hold an inclusive vision has yet taken in our society.

The reference to this possibility provides an occasion for warning against a too optimistic view of the immediate relevance of the ideal of spirit-centered wholeness. Soleri is himself a fine embodiment of the spiritual ideal. His vision is extraordinarily comprehensive. It has led him to a relatively holistic style of personal life. Nevertheless, there remains a tension between the relative embodiment of the vision now and the price that must be paid if the vision is to be more fully realized. The quality of life which the city would make possible for those who lived in it cannot be enjoyed by those who are trying to build it. For them, sacrifice is necessary, including a sacrifice of wholeness.

Apart from these examples of how the comprehensive vision can express itself in ways that are beneficial simultaneously for the self and for the world, spiritual existence ordered to a holistic view is compatible with innumerable programs of self-improvement. Physical exercise, sensitivity training, consciousness-raising, various Yogas, and many other disciplines are available and appropriate alongside traditional disciplines of study. Insofar as wholeness means the cultivation of all our potentialities, there is no limit to how far spirit-centered wholeness can go.

There is, however, a profound difference between spirit-centered wholeness and the wholeness described earlier. That wholeness involves fullness of presence and spontaneity. If one practices some new discipline it is not out of a need to be more inclusive but simply because at some point one finds that an attractive thing to do. Spirit-centered wholeness loses that spontaneity as it consciously orders and controls the personality. The wholeness it works to attain is not a given received by those who refuse its disruption but a conscious integration of many disciplined aspects of personal existence. Something precious has been lost.

5. The possibility and advantage of Spirit-centered wholeness

Given the negative character of this loss of spontaneity, it is not surprising that disciplines have developed for recovering it. The most serious and effective of these come from Zen. Zen can offer itself as an ideal lying beyond spirit-centered wholeness. The point here is that it is a different ideal and one which is realized through the overcoming of spirit. It is eminently appropriate for further investigation and evaluation, and, in my view, there are ways in which we may eventually move to some integration of the Buddhist realization of Emptiness and spirit-centered wholeness. But that lies beyond this paper. Here we will consider the fulfillment of spirit-centered wholeness in Spirit-centered wholeness. This introduced the complex and controversial issue of the divine element in the world.

What makes spirit-centered wholeness unsatisfactory for many of us is its style of control. Because spirit-centered persons reflect about all aspects of their existence and how to order them, they are in position consciously to leave them undeveloped or to develop them in one direction or another. This can lead to a sort of self-manipulation or even self-construction that removes us a long way from the naturalness that is associated with real wholeness. It seems to turn the human being into an artificial product. It expresses the extreme extension of the mechanical world view, with the spirit placed in the position of the artificer. It is of a piece with human efforts to "master" all of nature and shape it to our will.

However, spirit-centered people have another option. Without abandoning their ability to think about this whole range of issues and to act according to their conclusions, they can turn from the stance of control to that of trusting service. (This depends on acknowledging there to be something they do not control which is worthy of trust.)

The two attitudes can be illustrated at many points. Some doctors think of the human body as a machine. When it malfunctions, they mend it. Other doctors see the human body as a mysterious and wonderful system which includes the power of self-healing and growth. When this power is blocked or inhibited, the doctor can intervene to remove obstacles to its working. But the doctor trusts and serves this healing power.

Similarly some psychotherapists see themselves as the source of the cure they seek. By their skill and knowledge they control the development of the patient. Other therapists believe that there is potentiality and power for health within the client or within the system of relations between the client and others. The therapist's task is so to act that this healing power becomes more effective.

The same alternative exists in relating to what is going on within one's own body and psyche. One may perceive this activity as in itself neutral and directionless, so that the transcendent self decides for it and controls it. Alternately one may see both body and psyche as embodying a tendency toward health growth. If one experiences life in this way, one may trust what is not within one's control and serve it.

The adoption of this latter attitude does not depend on the name given to that which one trusts and serves. One may call it Nature, or Life, or Creativity, or Eros, or Goddess. Here we will call it Spirit. What does matter is whether we believe that there is here a wisdom greater than our own which is worthy of our trust. If we do not, we will need to try to control events on the basis of our present understanding. If we do, we will be open to having our own understanding changed as we listen to the promptings of the Spirit.

If we do believe that there is trustworthy power and wisdom not in our control, the question of the right relation thereto becomes important. When this power is understood in certain ways, then passivity is encouraged. There is the idea, for example, that God is the potter and we are the clay. There is the notion of complete self-surrender. There is the slogan: Let go and let God. But the Spirit is not a force outside other forces to which other forces including the human spirit should be subordinated. It is a power which operates only in and through other powers, to empower, to enliven, and to direct. Passivity is the refusal, not the acceptance, of its gift. But the image of co-working also fails. That too requires two separate powers acting together. What we need is an active acceptance of life or power, an active responsiveness to the directivity it contains. This entails rigorous thinking and vigorous acting in the public world. The attitude of trust does not reduce energy with which we strive to realize our vision. But it does recognize the power that it trusts as at work everywhere even in those who oppose one's proposals, and it is open to the surprise that effective agents of the Spirit can be found in the most unlikely places.

Trusting the Spirit does not lead one to regard the "wisdom of the body" as infallible. But it does lead one to attend to the body and to take seriously what one hears when one does so. This may lead to the same regimen of diet, exercise, relaxation, and sleep that follows from the attitude of control. But it may not. One may learn of somewhat different needs if one listens to one's own very particular body. And in any case the relation will be different. One will not be imposing on one's body what one has learned from other sources is good for the body. One will instead be guided by the body to give the body the chance to do what it wants and needs. Even when the requirement of the spirit necessitates the subordination of the body's claims, the denial of those claims will be with love and tenderness.

A similar change occurs at the level of spirit itself. The importance of the vision that orients all of life to purposes that are wider than oneself is not reduced. But it is now recognized that this vision itself is the gift of the Spirit. There is therefore a subtle but important shift in commitment. Instead of being committed finally to the vision and its implications for action, the commitment is directed toward the One who gave the vision.

This does not mean that one ceases to believe in the vision. One is no less sure that the people should be liberated or that the threat of war should be removed. But one does know that the vision is not absolute. The One who gave the vision can also enlarge and deepen it. In short, one is open to new insight and imagination. One will put oneself into those situations and those attitudes in which such new understanding is most likely to emerge. One will not suppose that apart from the gift of the Spirit one can produce them. One's own vision is not under one's control.

The attitude of trust in Spirit conduces to wholeness. It also makes the quest for wholeness less urgent. If one trusts the Spirit, one knows that one is all right as one is. One does not have to become whole in order to be all right as one is. One does not have to become whole in order to be all right. One is free to seek wholeness in service to the Spirit that makes for wholeness because there is no need to become whole.

Trust in divine power is not a new idea in relation to the idea of spirit. Indeed, it is quickly suggested by the term, and most of the heroes of the spirit in the past have believed in God and trusted. The rise of spirit in history was closely related to belief in God, and in the writings of St. Paul it is often difficult to distinguish spirit and Spirit. Unfortunately, for the most part, the way Spirit has been understood has not encouraged the quest for wholeness. It has more often encouraged the warfare of spirit with flesh. In spite of the differences between wholeness centered in Spirit and wholeness centered in spirit, the former remains a form of the latter. Wholeness centered in Spirit is wholeness centered in the spirit that lives by trust in Spirit. Through that trust Spirit itself becomes the center, but in doing so it does not set spirit aside. It fulfills it.

Conclusions

Wholeness centered in spirit is not the only ideal appropriate to our time, but it is an important one. It cannot be attained by the expansion of a wholeness that lacks spirit. It can only be realized by a transformation and enrichment of the life of spirit. That requires that the vision out of which spirit orders human existence become inclusive and that we find ways to overcome the tensions between the fulfillment of the self and the needs of the whole. Finally, to overcome the centrality of control with its accompanying loss of spontaneity and presence, it is desirable that spirit identify Spirit and trust it.

Author Index

Subject Index

Studies in the Psychology of Religion

1. James Gollnick, **Dreams in the Psychology of Religion**
2. H. Newton Malony, Michele Papen-Daniels, Howard Clinebell, Spirit-Centered Wholeness: Beyond the Psychology of Self
3. J. Harley Chapman, **Jung's Three Theories of Religious Experience**